Diabetes

Diabetes

John A. Colwell, MD, PhD

Professor of Medicine
Director, Diabetes Center
Medical University of South Carolina
Charleston, South Carolina

HANLEY & BELFUS
An Imprint of Elsevier

HANLEY & BELFUS
An Imprint of Elsevier

The Curtis Center
Independence Square West
Philadelphia, Pennsylvania 19106

Note to the reader: Although the information in this book has been carefully reviewed for correctness of dosage and indications, neither the author nor the publisher can accept any legal responsibility for any errors or omissions that may be made. Neither the publisher nor the author make any warranty, expressed or implied, with respect to the material contained herein. Before prescribing any drug, the reader must review the manufacturer's current product information (package inserts) for accepted indications, absolute dosage recommendations, and other information pertinent to the safe and effective use of the product described.

Library of Congress Control Number: 2003100108

DIABETES: HOT TOPICS

ISBN 1-56053-562-8

Printed in the United States of America

Last digit is the print number: 9 8 7 6 5 4 3 2 1

Contents

DEDICATION

I dedicate this book to my wife of 48 years, Jane. She has endured my many hours of preparation with tremendous insight, patience, understanding, and humor. I thank my role model and original mentor, my father, Dr. Arthur R. Colwell, Sr. He transmitted a genuine understanding and enthusiasm for my work and for the incredible challenges of dealing with people affected by diabetes and its complications. I also thank my colleagues and staff of the Diabetes Center at the Medical University of South Carolina and the many loyal and responsive patients with diabetes whom I have had the privilege to care for over the years. Finally, this book would not have been possible without the superb administrative and secretarial talents of Janice Lane.

Preface

In less than 10 years there has been a revolution in the standards of care for people with type 1 and type 2 diabetes. For 70 years after the discovery of insulin, debate raged in the scientific community about the benefits and risks of intensive control of the blood glucose to prevent complications in people with diabetes. The Diabetes Control and Complications Trial (DCCT), a landmark prospective, randomized trial, demonstrated conclusive and remarkable reduction in the risks for progression of retinopathy, nephropathy, and neuropathy in type 1 diabetes. The DCCT was followed by another seminal trial, the United Kingdom Prospective Diabetes Study (UKPDS), which revealed comparable results in people with type 2 diabetes. Suddenly physicians, other health professionals, and diabetic patients were faced with the necessity of achieving the best possible blood glucose control without severe hypoglycemia.

A second series of exciting advances rapidly changed the approach to prevention of major cardiovascular events in people with diabetes. Epidemiologic studies have shown that people with type 2 diabetes have at least a 2- to 4-fold increased risk of a major cardiovascular event than comparable nondiabetic people. A person with type 2 diabetes has the same risk of dying from a heart attack as a nondiabetic person who has already had one heart attack. Fortunately, a series of important clinical trials has shown definitive reduction in cardiovascular risk by intensive management of blood pressure, lipids, albuminuria, and the prothrombotic state that is found in type 2 diabetes. Other risk factors are under intensive study, and major future advances in therapy are anticipated.

The goal of this book is to provide the latest information for primary care health professionals about how to manage diabetes mellitus and its many complications. An evidence-based approach is used to develop methods of intensive management. Both type 1 and type 2 diabetes are covered in detail, with emphasis on type 2 as the most common challenge to the practicing health professional. The first section of the book deals with the scope and impact of diabetes and with the new criteria for its classification and diagnosis. Type 1 diabetes and its major complications of retinopathy, nephropathy, and neuropathy are described, and the latest guidelines for care are provided. The core of this section is a modern, practical approach to intensive management of people with type 1 diabetes. The team approach to glycemic regulation and to the prevention of progression of complications is emphasized. Evidence from major prospective collaborative clinical trials is liberally utilized.

The second major section of the book covers type 2 diabetes and its complications and presents a therapeutic approach based on the pathophysiology and natural history of the disease. Early recognition of people who are at high risk for type 2 diabetes or have components of metabolic syndrome (insulin resistance syndrome) is addressed as a key challenge. Early recognition of such people can result in preventing or delaying the onset of type 2 diabetes and its many complications. Intensive management of type 2 diabetes is viewed as a multifactorial challenge. Thus, whereas intensive glycemic control is a major goal that can be accomplished in the majority of patients, it may actually be more important to use aggressive measures to delay the progression of cardiovascular complications, which account for the majority of the staggering costs, morbidity, and mortality from diabetes. Fortunately, solid evidence supports intensive management of blood pressure, lipids, nephropathy, prothrombotic state, and congestive heart failure in type 2 diabetes. Methods to achieve intensive glycemic regulation and cardiovascular risk prevention are clearly provided.

Throughout the text, there is liberal use of tables, figures, and key points that summarize each section. Challenging and interesting cases of patients with type 1 and type 2 diabetes are presented. The book concludes with a discussion of myths about diabetes and an overall summary of intensive management of type 1 and type 2 diabetes mellitus.

I sincerely hope that this book will be valuable for all health professionals who regularly deal with the many challenges of providing modern care for patients with diabetes and its complications.

John A. Colwell, M.D., Ph.D.

What's Hot in Diabetes

Historical Perspective

For many years, physicians who dealt with diabetic patients were often passive in their treatment strategies. There were reasons for this. Many type 1 diabetics were very difficult to manage, alternating between hyper- and hypoglycemia, and progressing with complications of visual impairment, renal insufficiency, and neurologic disabilities. Assessment of results was crude, and action steps were based upon urine glucose levels or on occasional blood glucose determinations done during infrequent office visits. Inaction often was the result.

Concomitantly, the much larger population with type 2 diabetes did not do well. There were limited choices for drug therapy—older insulin preparations which were antigenic and poorly timed for the demands of the disease, and an oral agent formulary which was limited to the sulfonylurea drug class. Huge doses of insulin were needed for glycemic control and some questions had been raised about cardiotoxicity of sulfonylurea drugs. There was little recognition of the input of dyslipidemia, hypertension, or a prothrombotic state to the cardiovascular complications of type 2 diabetes. Further, there was a paucity of effective drugs to address these critical cardiovascular risk factors.

The picture was clouded by a tendency for apathy on the part of the patients. Physicians spoke of "noncompliance," while patients were not certain what to comply with or how to do it effectively. To many physicians and patients, management of diabetes was a nightmare. Fatalism prevailed.

All of this changed dramatically in the last decade. A proactive climate now prevails. Evidence-based guidelines have emerged, and the tools for effectively dealing with type 1 and type 2 diabetes and preventing progression of complications are now generally available. The key issue now is translation of the findings of this revolution in diabetic care to positive action by physicians and patients.

Type 1 Diabetes

As a result of a landmark study, the Diabetes Control and Complications Trial (DCCT), there has been a revolution in care for people with type 1 diabetes. It was conclusively demonstrated that progression of microvascular complications, particularly retinopathy, can be delayed or prevented by intensive control of blood glucose. This has now been made possible by major advances in monitoring glucose excursions, estimating total glycemic exposure by measuring HbA1c, and in treatment using newly designed human insulins, either by insulin pump or by injections. It was clear in the DCCT and confirmed as its findings were translated into practice that a team approach with a physician, a nurse specially trained in diabetic management, and a nutritionist is the way to accomplish this degree of diabetic control.

Future therapeutic developments include perfection of techniques for transplantation of islet cells and development of a closed loop system which would measure glucose concentrations and deliver the proper insulin dosage by an automated pump. New methods of giving insulin without requiring an injection, such as inhaled insulin, show promise.

Finally, major headway has been made in preventing the vascular complications which have traditionally affected type 1 diabetics. In particular, monitoring of small amounts of albumin in the urine (microalbuminuria) will identify people who may progress to renal insufficiency. It is clear that this progression may be delayed or stopped by therapy with angiotensin-converting enzyme inhibitors (ACE-I) or receptor blockers (ARB). In an analogous fashion, aggressive treatment of elevated blood pressure, with a new guideline of B.P. $\leq 130/80$ mm/hg, will delay or prevent progression not only of renal insufficiency, but also of retinopathy. This can be accomplished in most patients, often with combinations of newly developed agents: ACE-I (or ARB), calcium channel blockers, cardiospecific beta blockers, and thiazides.

Type 2 Diabetes

A critical issue in type 2 diabetes is the steady increase in prevalence over the past decade, particularly in developed countries. There has been an alarming increase in numbers of obese individuals and the choice of a sedentary lifestyle. It is now clear that type 2 diabetes is caused by a combination of insulin resistance and progressive insulin deficiency, and therapy must be directed at both defects. Exciting studies have now demonstrated that intensive lifestyle changes, including a regular exercise conditioning program and modest weight reduction (5–10%), will delay the onset of type 2 diabetes in those with impaired glucose tolerance. Specific methods to accomplish this, as was done in the research trials, are now widely promoted. Translation to the real world will be difficult.

One of the most exciting developments in diabetes is the general acceptance by the medical community that a metabolic syndrome (previously called Syndrome X or the Insulin Resistance Syndrome) usually precedes and accompanies clinical diabetes. This syndrome has the essential components of impaired glucose tolerance (or frank diabetes), centripetal obesity, hypertension, elevated plasma triglyceride, and low plasma HDL cholesterol levels in variable combinations. Other vascular risk factors may be present, such as microalbuminuria and decreased fibrinolytic activity. A focus on prevention of future cardiovascular events in these people who often have "mild" diabetes has dramatically changed our therapeutic strategies, very early in the course of diabetes mellitus.

As a result of another landmark study, The United Kingdom Prospective Diabetes Study (UKPDS), we now recognize that type 2 diabetes is a progressive disease. Beta-cell function gradually deteriorates over time. Insulin resistance may rise, secondary to hyperglycemia ("glucose toxicity"). Aggressive drug therapy is needed—with newly approved oral agents that will address the dual defects of deficient insulin secretion (third generation sulfonylureas, meglitinides) and insulin resistance (thiazolidinediones). Metformin acts on a third physiologic component of uncontrolled diabetes: increased hepatic glucose production. We can now limit dietary carbohydrate breakdown by alpha-glucosidase inhibitors. Thus, before insulin is needed, one can often control glycemia by new drug combinations that address specific pathophysiologic alterations in type 2 diabetes. When insulin is required, we now have newly developed products that will address the issue of increased hepatic glucose output during the overnight fasting period. Combinations of oral drugs with insulin are proving to be acceptable strategies. With this multifactorial aggressive approach to hyperglycemia, the UKPDS demonstrated that progression of microvascular events could be delayed in type 2 diabetes.

In spite of all of this, people with type 2 diabetes usually die from cardiovascular events, and they have the same very high risk for myocardial infarction as nondiabetics who have already had a heart attack! The good news is that additional prospective collaborative trials have conclusively shown that major risk reductions in cardiovascular events can be achieved by intensive control of blood pressure, lipid abnormalities, and the prothrombotic state characteristic of type 2 diabetes. Thus, combination therapy for hypertension, as in type 1 diabetics, will lower the risk for cardiovascular events and progression of retinopathy and nephropathy. Statin therapy has revolutionized cholesterol-lowering strategies, and studies continue to support this treatment in diabetics of all ages, either gender, and as a primary or secondary prevention approach. Fibrate therapy has been shown to decrease risk for cardiac events in diabetics with low HDL cholesterol, and many studies support the use of low-dose aspirin for the prothrombotic state, which is frequently present.

Exciting research indicates that other potentially treatable risk markers are present in diabetes. Atherosclerosis is now recognized as an inflammatory disease, and the plasma level c-reactive protein (CRP), as determined by a highly sensitive new assay, has proven to be a cardiovascular risk marker. Studies are underway to determine if drugs which lower CRP levels (e.g., aspirin or nonsteroidal anti-inflammatory drugs) will decrease cardiovascular events. Homocysteine metabolism is occasionally altered in diabetes, and prospective trials are underway to determine if lowering plasma levels with folic acid, B_6, or B_{12} will prevent cardiovascular events.

Thus, there is more than a hotplate full of topics in type 1 and type 2 diabetes. Rather, consider a gigantic oven, with multiple shelves, nooks, and crannies in which a plethora of hot items are being baked at variable rates. In some areas, microwave speed has been achieved. The net effect is a body of new information which must be transmitted and understood by health care professionals in order to improve the lives of people with diabetes mellitus.

Scope and Impact of Diabetes in the U.S.

chapter
1

Prevalence

Diabetes mellitus is a chronic disorder that is seen with increasing frequency. Prevalence rises with age (Fig. 1). Approximately 20% (7 million) of people over age 65 have diabetes. In the United States, prevalence estimates are made by the Centers for Disease Control and Prevention and state health departments, using a yearly cross-sectional telephone survey. This method, the Behavioral Risk Factor Surveillance System (BRFSS), obtains a representative sample of each state's noninstitutionalized civilian residents, aged 18 years or older. Prevalence estimates of diagnosed diabetes by this system rose 50% in the 1990s, from 4.9% in 1990 to 6.5% in 1998 and 7.3% in 2000.[11] The census in the year 2000 estimated that there were about 196 million adults over the age of 18 in the U.S.[12,19] This figure suggests that there were at least 14 million adults with known diabetes in 2000. Epidemiologic surveys have generally shown that for every two people with known diabetes there is at least one person who has diabetes and does not know it.[4,5] Thus, approximately 10% of the adult population, or 20 million adults in the U.S., may have diabetes mellitus. The majority of these cases are type 2 diabetes. Finally, if one includes the 15.6% of adults who are estimated to have impaired glucose tolerance (IGT),[5] more than 25% of the U.S. population over the age of 18 has abnormal glucose metabolism.

The American Diabetes Association gives a more conservative estimate: 17 million people with diabetes in the U.S. with 11.1 million diagnosed and 5.9 million undiagnosed. An additional million people have a condition called "pre-diabetes," which is defined as either impaired glucose tolerance or impaired fasting glucose (IFG). These terms are described in Chapter 2. Whatever the true frequency, it is clear that diabetes is a major public health issue.[17]

This alarming increase in the prevalence of type 2 diabetes and pre-diabetes is accompanied by a comparable increase in the number of overweight (BMI $\geq$ 25kg/m^2) or obese (BMI $\geq$ 30kg/m^2) people.[10,11] In

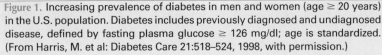

Figure 1. Increasing prevalence of diabetes in men and women (age ≥ 20 years) in the U.S. population. Diabetes includes previously diagnosed and undiagnosed disease, defined by fasting plasma glucose ≥ 126 mg/dl; age is standardized. (From Harris, M. et al: Diabetes Care 21:518–524, 1998, with permission.)

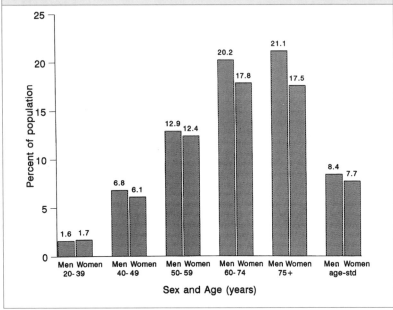

1991, 12.3% of the U.S. population was obese and 45% was overweight. These rates rose to 19.8% and 56.4%, respectively, by 2000. Thus, over 75% of the U.S. adult population was overweight in 2000, and over 25% had altered glucose metabolism. Similar trends are seen in people under 18 years of age, and type 2 diabetes is now recognized with increased frequency in overweight or obese children and adolescents.[2,14]

The prevalence of type 2 diabetes is higher among African Americans, Hispanic Americans, Mexican Americans, and Native Born Americans compared with Caucasians.[4] Increases in the U.S. population of some of these ethnic groups have contributed to the overall rise in prevalence of diabetes in the U.S. in the past decade. Thus, the trends shown in older surveys (Fig. 1) are likely to be magnified with modern data.

Estimates of the prevalence of type 1 diabetes in the U.S. are about 1.7 per 1000 people aged 1–19, and about 1.2 per 1000 people of all ages. In 2000, this suggests close to 350,000 people with type 1 diabetes in the U.S.[9] Other estimates suggest that the prevalence is about 0.3% of adults over the age of 30, or close to 500,000 older people with type 1 diabetes in 2000.[7] In any case, relative to type 2 diabetes, type 1 is a rare disease and probably accounts for less than 5% of the entire population of close to 20 million people with diabetes in the U.S. However, there are about 30,000 new cases of type 1 diabetes each year, and it is said to be the most frequent chronic childhood disease.[8]

Undiagnosed Type 2 Diabetes

Convincing information from analyses of the National Health and Nutrition Surveys (NHANES III) indicates that undiagnosed type 2 diabetes and IGT are highly prevalent in the U.S. population.[4] Prevalence is 14–20% in those over 50 years of age. Retinopathy is present in approximately 20% of type 2 diabetic patients at the time of diagnosis and is estimated to start at least 4–7 years before the clinical diagnosis is made.[6] Using the older diagnostic criteria of fasting plasma glucose $\geq$ 140 mg/dl (instead of the presently accepted $\geq$126 mg/dl), it was estimated that the onset of type 2 diabetes probably occurred about 12 years before diagnosis. This period is not benign. The prevalence of macrovascular disease at this stage is the same as in diagnosed diabetes, and the rates of coronary heart disease in both diagnosed and undiagnosed people with diabetes are at least twice that of nondiabetic people. Similar data are found for mortality.[3]

Cardiovascular risk factors are usually present in excess before the diagnosis of type 2 diabetes is made. In the NHANES II analysis, prior to the diagnosis of type 2 diabetes, the prevalence of hypertension was 61%; hypercholesterolemia, 49%; LDL cholesterol > 130 mg/dl, 62%; elevated plasma triglycerides, 28%; and obesity, 50% (men) and 82% (women).

Using the older criteria (FPG $\geq$ 140 mg/dl) for the diagnosis of diabetes, it was estimated that 50% of the type 2 diabetic population was not diagnosed. This figure falls to about 33% when the newer criteria of FPG $\geq$126 mg/dl are used. Whichever criterion is used, it is evident that undiagnosed type 2 diabetes is a major public health problem.[5,10,17]

Health Resource Utilization

In 1997, total direct and indirect expenditures attributable to diabetes mellitus and its complications were $98 billion.[1] Direct medical expenditures were $44.1 billion, including $7.7 billion for diabetes and acute glycemic care, $11.8 billion for the excessive prevalence of related chronic complications, and $24.6 billion for the excessive prevalence of general medical conditions. The majority of these expenditures were for inpatient care (62%), followed by outpatient services (25%) and nursing home care (13%). The indirect costs of $54.1 billion included $17.0 billion resulting from premature mortality and $37.1 billion from disability. Total medical expenditures borne by people with diabetes totaled $77.7

billion, or $10,071 per capita each year, compared with $2,669/year for people without diabetes. This total equaled about 8% of all expenditures for health services in 1997.

In 1997, people with diabetes accounted for 13.87 million days in the hospital, 30.3 million physician visits, and 3.55 million emergency room encounters. Close to 50 million medications were dispensed for the care of diabetes. People with diabetes lost an average of 8.3 days from work each year, a fivefold increase above the mean of 1.7 days/year for people without diabetes. Even these staggering statistics represent a major underestimate of the true costs of this disease, for they do not include data from federal hospitals, undiagnosed diabetics, or people with IGT. Further, evidence suggests serious undercoding of diabetes as a diagnosis on hospital records and on death certificates.[17] The economic burden is obviously enormous.

There is some good news, however. A slight decline in direct costs (from $45.2 billion to $44.1 billion) occurred between 1992 and 1997. This decline was in the face of the increasing prevalence of diabetes and a steady, modest increase in the rate of inflation, both of which should have increased direct costs. The decrease in direct costs was most likely due to a dramatic decrease in the mean length of hospital stay and to a shift in site of service to the outpatient arena. In 1992, 20.2 million inpatient days were attributed to diabetes;[13] this figure decreased about 31% to 13.9 million days in 1997. Inpatient costs decreased from $37.2 billion in 1992 to $27.5 billion in 1997. Concomitantly, there was a large increase in outpatient expenditures and home health care for people with diabetes. Intensive glycemic regulation in type 1 and in type 2 diabetes was shown to delay progression of microvascular complications at a reasonable cost.[16,18]

The most encouraging news, however, is the constellation of major medical advances in the care for people with diabetes and its complications. We now have excellent scientific evidence, primarily from recently completed large scale controlled intervention trials, that intensive treatment of glycemia, blood pressure, lipids, and albuminuria delays the onset or prevent the major microvascular and macrovascular complications of diabetes. Low-dose aspirin therapy significantly decreases the incidence of cardiovascular events in type 2 diabetics and in type 1 diabetics with increased cardiovascular risk. Furthermore, the onset of the disorder can be substantially delayed by lifestyle changes or medication in people who are at high risk for the development of diabetes mellitus. Thus, intensive medical therapy has a tremendous potential to decrease the enormous costs of diabetes and its complications. The present challenge is to translate this information into the real world of diabetes care.

Mortality

A representative cohort of 14,374 adults (aged 25–74) was identified in NHANES I in 1971–1975 and followed for 22 years.[3] Death certificates were examined to determine cause of death in diabetic and nondiabetic subjects. Diabetes accounted for 5.1% of the cohort but 10.6% of the deaths. Age-adjusted mortality rates were 57% higher in diabetic men than in women and 27% higher in African Americans than in Caucasians with diabetes. Mortality was highest for insulin-treated patients and those with diabetes for 15 years or longer. Heart disease was listed most frequently—on 69.5% of the death certificates for people with diabetes. The excessive mortality, however, was not completely explained by differences in risk factors for heart disease. A twofold excessive risk can be attributed to other factors operative in the diabetic state. Similar findings were reported by Stamler in a 12-year analysis of diabetic men in the Multiple Risk Factor Intervention Trial (MRFIT).[15]

Thus, despite underreporting of diabetes as a contributing factor on death certificates, mortality rates are substantially higher in people with diabetes compared with nondiabetics. Rates are higher in men than in women and in African Americans than in Caucasians. Life expectancy is markedly diminished. The majority of deaths are related to heart disease, suggesting that increased attention to management of cardiovascular risk factors can decrease the mortality rate and increase life expectancy for people with diabetes. These predictions are now strongly supported by prospective randomized trials directed at management of a variety of cardiovascular risk markers, including hypertension, dyslipidemia, albuminuria, nephropathy, and the prothrombotic tendency that often occurs in diabetes.

Key Points: Scope and Impact of Diabetes in the U.S.

- Prevalence of diagnosed diabetes has risen from 4.9% in 1990 to 7.3% in 2000.
- There are approximately 12–14 million adults with known diabetes. Prevalence rises with increasing age.
- An additional 6–7 million adults have diabetes but do not know it.
- When people with IGT are included, over 25% of the adult population in the U.S. has abnormal glucose metabolism.
- Type 1 diabetes is present in less than 1 million people in the U.S.
- In 1997, expenditures attributable to diabetes were $98 billion.
- Total medical expenditures by people with diabetes in 1997 were in excess of $10,000/year, about 4 times the expenditures for people without diabetes.

Key Points (*Continued*)

↪ People with diabetes lose about 8.3 days from work each year, 5 times the days lost by those without diabetes.

↪ A shift from hospital to outpatient-based care resulted in a decrease in direct costs for diabetes between 1992 and 1997, despite increased prevalence of the disease.

↪ Major cardiovascular risk factors are usually present in excess before the diagnosis of type 2 diabetes as well as during the course of the disease.

↪ Major advances in preventive measures directed at the complications of micro and macrovascular disease will lead to reduced costs of diabetes in the future, if translated into usual diabetes care.

References

1. American Diabetes Association: Economic consequences of diabetes mellitus in the U.S. in 1997. Diabetes Care 21:296–309, 1998.
2. American Diabetes Association: Type 2 diabetes in children and adolescents. Diabetes Care 23:381–389, 2000.
3. Gu K, Cowie CC, Harris MI: Mortality in adults with and without diabetes in a national cohort of the U.S. population, 1971–1993. Diabetes Care 21:1138–1145, 1998.
4. Harris MI, Flegal KM, Cowie CC, et al: Prevalence of diabetes, impaired fasting glucose, and impaired glucose tolerance in U.S. adults. Diabetes Care 21:518–524, 1998.
5. Harris, MI: Undiagnosed NIDDM: Clinical and public health issues. Diabetes Care 16:642–652, 1993.
6. Harris MI, Klein R, Welborn TA, et al: Onset of NIDDM occurs at least 4–7 yr before clinical diagnosis. Diabetes 15:815–819, 1992.
7. Harris MI, Robbins DC: Prevalence of adult-onset IDDM in the U.S. population. Diabetes Care 17:1337–1340, 1994.
8. Karvonen M, Viik-Kajander M, Motchanova E, et al: Incidence of childhood type 1 diabetes worldwide. Diabetes Care 23:1516–1526, 2000.
9. LaPorte RE, Matsushima M, Chang, YF: Prevalence and incidence of insulin-dependent diabetes. In Diabetes in America, 2nd ed. National Institutes of Health, National Institute of Diabetes and Digestive and Kidney Disease. NIH Publication No. 95–1468. 1995, pp 37–45.
10. Mokdad AH, Ford ES, Bowman BA, et al: Diabetes trends in the U.S.: 1990–1998. Diabetes Care 23:1278–1283, 2000.
11. Mokdad AH, Bowman BA, Ford ES, et al: The continuing epidemics of obesity and diabetes in the United States. JAMA 286:1195–1200, 2001.
12. Perry, MJ, Mackun, PJ, et al: Population change and distribution 1990 to 2000. In United States Census 2000. Washington, DC, U.S. Census Bureau, 2001, pp 2–7.
13. Rubin RJ, Altman WM, Mendelson DN: Health care expenditures for people with diabetes mellitus, 1992. JCE & M 78:809A–809F, 1994.
14. Sinha R, Fisch G, Teague B, et al: Prevalence of impaired glucose tolerance among children and adolescents with marked obesity. N Engl J Med 346:802–810, 2002.

15. Stamler J, Vaccaro O, Neaton JD, et al: Diabetes, other risk factors, and 12-yr cardiovascular mortality for men screened in the multiple risk factor intervention trial. Diabetes Care 16:434–444, 1993.

16. The Diabetes Control and Complications Trial Research Group: Resource utilization and costs of care in the diabetes control and complications trial. Diabetes Care 18:1468–1478, 1995.

17. Tokuhata GK, Miller W, Digon E, Hartman T: Diabetes mellitus: An underestimated public health problem. J. Chron Dis 28:23–35, 1975.

18. UKPDS: Cost effectiveness of an intensive blood glucose control policy in patients with type 2 diabetes economic analysis alongside randomised controlled trial (UKPDS 41). BMJ 320:1373–1378, 2000.

19. U.S. Census Bureau: Profiles of general demographic characteristics 2000. In United States Census 2000. Washington, DC, U.S. Census Bureau, 2001, Table DPI, p 1.

Classification, Diagnosis, and Screening for Diabetes

chapter
2

History

The classification and diagnosis of diabetes used in the U.S. were developed by the National Diabetes Data Group (NDDG) in 1979.[6] Because of the development of new knowledge, the American Diabetes Association established an International Expert Committee in May, 1995, to review the scientific literature since 1979 and decide whether changes were warranted. The Committee developed a report, sought wide input, made revisions based on consensus, and published a new classification and diagnosis scheme.[8]

Classification of Diabetes

The new classification has the following critical features:
- The terms insulin-dependent or non–insulin-dependent (IDDM or NIDDM) are eliminated. The terms are confusing and based on treatment rather than the preferred factor—cause (Table 1).
- Type 1 and type 2 diabetes are retained, using Arabic rather than Roman numerals. Type 1 diabetes may be due to an autoimmune process or unknown causes. Subclasses, therefore, are autoimmune and idiopathic. An autoimmune process is suggested by the presence of islet cell, glutamic acid decarboxylase (GAD), or insulin autoantibodies in plasma.
- Type 2 diabetes is the most prevalent form and results from insulin resistance plus insulin secretory defects.
- Impaired glucose tolerance (IGT) is retained. A new term, impaired fasting glucose (IFG) is defined as fasting glucose ≥ 110 and < 126 mg/dl.
- Gestational diabetes mellitus (GDM) is retained.
- The severity of the metabolic abnormality may progress, regress, or stay the same.
- Many diabetic people may not easily fit into a single class. For

9

example, GDM may evolve into type 1 diabetes or diabetes after glucocorticoids or thiazides, regress, and return later.
- The incidence and prevalence of type 2 diabetes in children and adolescents is increasing. These patients often come from ethnic groups at high risk for diabetes, are usually overweight, and may have a strong family history of diabetes. Diagnostic criteria are the same as in adults.

Diagnostic Criteria

Diabetes Mellitus

There are three ways to diagnose diabetes:
1. Symptoms of diabetes with a casual (any time of the day) plasma glucose ≥200 mg/dl.
2. Fasting plasma glucose (FPG) ≥ 126 mg/dl on at least two occasions. Fasting = no caloric intake for at least 8 hr.
3. 2 hour plasma/glucose (PG) ≥ 200 mg/dl after 75 gm of oral glucose in water oral glucose tolerance test (OGTT).

Impaired Glucose Tolerance

Diagnostic test: 75 gm glucose orally

Time	Plasma glucose (mg/dl)
Fasting	< 120 mg/dl
2 hour	140–200 mg/dl

TABLE 1. Etiologic Classification of Diabetes
1. Type 1 (Beta cell destruction, usually leading to insulin deficiency)
• Immune-mediated
• Idiopathic
2. Type 2 (may range from predominantly insulin resistance with relative insulin deficiency to a predominantly insulin secretion defect, with insulin resistance).
3. Other specific types
• Genetic defects of beta cell function
• Genetic defects in insulin action
• Diseases of the exocrine pancreas
• Endocrinopathies
• Drug or chemical-induced
• Infections
• Uncommon focus of immune-mediated diabetes
• Genetic syndromes sometimes associated with diabetes
• Others
4. Gestational diabetes mellitus (GDM)

Gestational Diabetes Mellitus (GDM)[2]

Screening test: 50 gm oral glucose load, with 1 hour value ≥ 140mg/dl. The ADA recommends that the test be done between weeks 24 and 28 of pregnancy. The American College of Obstetrics and Gynecology (ACOG) recommends that all pregnant patients be screened and that the 1-hour value of 130 (90% sensitivity) or 140 mg/dl (80% sensitivity) be used as the threshold for diagnostic testing.[1] According to the ADA guidelines, testing is optional in low-risk groups: age < 25 years, normal body weight, no family history of diabetes, and not a member of an ethnic/racial group with a high prevalence of diabetes (Hispanic, African-American, Asian, Native American).

Diagnostic test: 100 gm glucose orally (if screening test is abnormal)

Time fasting	Plasma glucose (mg/dl)
	105
1 hr	190
2 hr	165
3 hr	145

Diagnosis of GDM: Any 2 of the 4 plasma glucose values meet or exceed above values.

Hemoglobin A1c as a Diagnostic Test

Pro: (1) Has a frequency distribution like FPG or 2-hour PG.

(2) Studies have established a level above which the likelihood of developing retinopathy and nephropathy increases dramatically. This level is approximately 6.0%.

Con: (1) Many different methods; limited standardization; limited world-wide availability.

(2) Imperfectly correlated with FPG, 2-hr PG.

Conclusion: HbA1c is not recommended as a diagnostic test at present.

Pre-diabetes

A new condition; pre-diabetes, was defined by the ADA in 2002. A person with IGT or impaired fasting glucose (IFG: fasting glucose of 110–125 mg/dl) is now defined as having pre-diabetes. Such people are at high risk for developing diabetes in the next decade and have an increased risk for coronary heart disease. The ADA has estimated that about 12 million people in the U.S. have pre-diabetes.

Screening for Type 2 Diabetes

Principles that guide the decision to use screening procedures in asymptomatic people include the following:[3]

1. Discovery of a disease that represents an important health problem and imposes a significant burden on the population.
2. An understanding of the natural history of the disease.
3. Recognition of a preclinical, asymptomatic stage at which the disease may be diagnosed.
4. Acceptable and reliable tests to detect the preclinical stage of the disease.
5. Evidence that treatment after early detection yields benefits superior to those obtained when treatment is delayed.
6. Reasonable costs of case finding and treatment, balanced in relation to overall health expenditures, facilities, and resources to treat newly diagnosed cases.
7. Continuation of a systematic ongoing process, not merely an isolated effort.

For diabetes, conditions 1–4 are met. Successful screening in an outpatient clinic has been shown.[5] Two recent reports have shown that the time of onset of diabetes can be delayed by intensive lifestyle modification[4,9] or metformin therapy.[4] These studies suggest that condition 5 is met. Evidence is less convincing, however, that screening is cost effective or is carried out as a systematic, ongoing process in most environments. Accordingly, the ADA has recommended that screening of high-risk individuals be considered by health care providers at 3-year intervals, beginning at age 45.[3] The major risk factors for type 2 diabetes are shown in Table 2.

If multiple risk factors are present, screening should be carried out at a younger age and more frequently. In high-risk children, screening should be done every 2 years, starting at age 10 (or at puberty, if it occurs at a younger age). Recent studies indicate that these guidelines should be adjusted to include screening under the age of 10 in obese children. Among 55 obese children referred to a pediatric obesity clinic, 25% of those aged 4–10 had IGT. Of 112 obese adolescents (ages 11–18 years), 21% had IGT and 4% had undiagnosed diabetes.[7]

TABLE 2. Major Risk Factors for Type 2 Diabetes
Family history of diabetes (i.e., parents or siblings with diabetes)
Overweight (BMI $\geq$ 25 kg/m^2)
Habitual physical inactivity
Race/ethnicity (e.g., African-Americans, Hispanic-Americans, Native Americans, Asian-Americans, and Pacific Islanders)
Previously identified IFG or IGT
Hypertension ($\geq$ 140/90 mmHg in adults)
HDL cholesterol $\leq$ 35 mg/dl and/or a triglyceride level $\geq$ 250 mg/dl
History of GDM or delivery of a baby weighing > 9 lb
Polycystic ovary syndrome

The best screening test is a fasting plasma glucose value, determined in a certified laboratory, after an overnight fast of at least 8 hours. It is important to recognize that fingerstick capillary glucose values are not accurate enough for screening purposes. An FPG ≥ 126 mg/dl should be repeated; if still elevated, the test indicates that diabetes is present. If FPG is < 126 mg/dl and suspicion of diabetes is high, an oral glucose tolerance should be performed. In view of the results of the Diabetes Prevention Program (DPP), an intervention trial done in overweight subjects with IGT, an increased use of oral glucose tolerance testing in people at high risk for type 2 diabetes should be done in the future. Intervention may then be indicated if IGT is found because studies have shown that onset of diabetes can be delayed by intensive diet and exercise[4,9] or metformin therapy.[4]

An interpretation of the screening test should be provided to the patient, and follow-up evaluation and treatment should be recommended. Although community screening programs may increase public awareness of diabetes, they are not recommended as a cost-effective approach to reduce the morbidity and mortality associated with diabetes in presumably healthy people.

Key Points: Classification, Diagnosis, and Screening for Diabetes

- In 1995, the classification of diabetes mellitus was changed, with the major categories being type 1 (immune-mediated or idiopathic) and type 2 diabetes mellitus.
- Diagnostic criteria for gestational diabetes mellitus (GDM), impaired glucose tolerance (IGT), impaired fasting glucose (IFG), and diabetes mellitus were updated.
- The major change was lowering the fasting plasma glucose from ≥ 140 mg/dl to ≥ 126 mg/dl for the diagnosis of diabetes mellitus.
- Pre-diabetes is defined by either IFG (110–125 mg/dl) or IGT.
- People with pre-diabetes are at a high risk for the development of diabetes and coronary heart disease.
- Screening for the presence of diabetes is best done by measuring the glucose concentration in a specimen of venous plasma, taken after an overnight (≥ 8 hours) fast.
- Fingerstick glucose testing is not accurate enough to use for screening.
- Screening should be confined to members of high-risk groups (Table 2)

Key Points (*Continued*)

↪ Two recent major studies have indicated that the onset of type 2 diabetes in people with IGT may be delayed by intensive lifestyle changes (diet and exercise). One study showed that metformin therapy was effective.

↪ These studies indicate that increased use of glucose tolerance testing in people at high risk for diabetes should be used in the future, because therapy may decrease the risk of diabetes.

References

1. American College of Obstetricians and Gynecologists: Gestational diabetes. Obstet Gynecol 98:525–538, 2001.
2. American Diabetes Association: Gestational diabetes. Diabetes Care 25:594–596, 2002.
3. Engelgau MM, Narayan KMV, Herman WH: Screening for type 2 diabetes. Diabetes 23:1563–1580, 2000.
4. Diabetes Prevention Program Research Group: Reduction in the incidence of Type 2 diabetes with lifestyle intervention or metformin. N Engl J Med 346:393–403, 2002.
5. Edelman D, Edwards LJ, Olsen MK, et al. Screening for diabetes in an outpatient clinic population. J Gen Intern Med 17:23–28, 2002.
6. National Diabetes Data Group: Classification and diagnosis of diabetes mellitus and other categories of glucose intolerance. Diabetes 28:1039–1057, 1979.
7. Sinha R, Fisch G, Teague B, et al: Prevalence of impaired glucose tolerance among children and adolescents with marked obesity. N Engl J Med 346:802–810, 2002.
8. The Expert Committee on the Diagnosis and Classification of Diabetes Mellitus: Report of the expert committee on the diagnosis and classification of diabetes mellitus. Diabetes Care 20:1183–1197,1997.
9. Tuomilehto J, Lindstrom J, Eriksson JG, et al: Prevention of type 2 diabetes mellitus by changes in lifestyle among subjects with impaired glucose tolerance. N Engl J Med 344:1343–1350, 2001.

Type 1 Diabetes

chapter
3

Pathogenesis

As noted in the section on classification of diabetes,[32] type 1 diabetes may be immune-mediated (type 1A) or idiopathic (type 1B). In either case, complete (or almost complete) loss of pancreatic beta cell function results in an absolute need for insulin therapy. The pathogenesis of immune-mediated destruction of the pancreatic beta cells has received the most attention, and is better understood than idiopathic loss of beta cell function.[5] Pathologically, it is characterized by degranulated beta cells, an inflammatory infiltrate, and preservation of the other pancreatic islet cells, such as the glucagon-secreting alpha cells or the somatostatin-producing delta cells. The inflammatory infiltrate is composed of lymphocytes (CD4 and CD8 cells), natural killer cells, and macrophages. Islet involvement may be variable, and the clinical course of islet destruction may be slow or rapid.

Autoantibodies in the plasma are predictive and diagnostic for type 1A diabetes. Autoantibodies to the pancreatic islets were the first to be described. Subsequently, other autoantibodies have been found, including antibodies to glutamic acid decarboxylase (GAD), insulin, and other islet cell antigens. Type 1 diabetes-associated autoantibodies have been recognized before the onset of clinical disease, and their presence indicates a high risk of developing type 1 diabetes. First-phase insulin release is often reduced, and hyperglycemia eventually occurs. Islet cell autoantibodies are present in at least 70–80% of people with newly diagnosed type 1 diabetes, and insulin autoantibodies are present in about 50%. As the disease progresses, titers of autoantibodies fall and may be undetectable with long-standing autoimmune type 1 diabetes. A relatively high incidence of other autoimmune diseases (thyroiditis, celiac disease, pernicious anemia, or Addison's disease) in people with type 1 diabetes supports the role of autoimmunity in the pathogenesis of the disease.

The components of the immune system that are primarily responsible for beta cell destruction are under study. Elaboration of the cytokine interleukin-1 (IL-1) is thought to be of pathogenetic importance. IL-1 inhibits insulin secretion and may be cytotoxic to the islets. Another cytokine, IL-6, is produced by beta cells and can stimulate the immune response, enhance insulitis, and result in beta cell destruction. In one model, it is hypothesized that viral infection of a beta cell increases release of cytokines and adhesion of leukocytes. The infected beta cell is susceptible to attack by antiviral cytotoxic CD8 lymphocytes. Macrophages in the islets are stimulated to produce cytokines and free radicals, increasing the cytotoxicity to the beta cells. Macrophages offer viral antigens to CD4 lymphocytes, which activate B lymphocytes to produce antiviral and anti–beta-cell antibodies. The process is obviously a complicated one with evolving concepts. The end product of virtually complete beta cell destruction leads to an absolute need for insulin therapy.

Genetics

Type 1 diabetes is a genetically determined disorder,[32] with an increased incidence in monozygotic twins and first-degree relatives of people with type 1 diabetes. Approximately 70% of monozygotic twins develop type 1 diabetes (with prolonged follow-up), and a first degree relative of a person with type 1 diabetes has approximately one chance in twenty (5% risk) of developing the disease (vs. 1:300 in the general population). The responsible genes are within the major histocompatability complex (MHC) located on chromosome 6 (also called the HLA locus). About 40% of the familial aggregation of autoimmune type 1 diabetes is explained by MHC genes, especially HLA class II molecules DQ and DR. Ninety-five percent of type 1 diabetics carry HLA D3, D4, or both compared with 45% of the general population. The presence of an aspartic acid residue at position 57 of the DQ β chain is protective for the development of type 1 diabetes. Clustering of long-term complications in families studied in the DCCT suggests that a genetic component contributes to vascular complications.[16]

Prevention of Type 1 Diabetes

An NIH-sponsored multicenter study, the Diabetes Prevention Trial 1 (DPT-1), explored the postulate that low-dose insulin, given subcutaneously, can delay or prevent type 1 diabetes in people at high risk. In DPT-1, however, injection of low-dose insulin did not change the rate of development of type 1 diabetes. A second arm of DPT-1 is exploring the postulate that orally administered insulin in people at moderate risk will delay or prevent the onset of type 1 diabetes.[3]

Natural History: Effect of Intensive Management

Insulin Secretion

Although the autoimmune process may result in complete beta cell destruction, this is not always the case, particularly in the early stages of the disease in youg adults. Before the development of serum c-peptide assays to assess insulin secretion in the presence of insulin therapy, clinicians had noted that people with type 1 diabetes who were treated with insulin may have a "honeymoon period," during which insulin requirements decrease, but metabolic control is maintained. Subsequently, after the development of the c-peptide assay, it was apparent that this phenomenon was due to the fact that basal and stimulated insulin secretion can be maintained for years in some people with type 1 diabetes.

The Diabetes Control and Complications Trial (DCCT) afforded a unique opportunity to study the natural history of type 1 diabetes longitudinally in a group 1441 of adolescents and adults with type 1 diabetes.[30] Furthermore, the design of the DCCT allowed analysis of the effect of standard vs. intensive glycemic management on pancreatic c-peptide secretion, a good index of insulin secretion.[22] Cross-sectional analyses of subjects screened for the trial demonstrated that a similar number of adults (45%) and adolescents (37%) with short diabetes duration (1–5 years) had evidence of insulin release with nutrient stimulation. The plasma levels of fasting and meal-stimulated c-peptide levels were closely correlated, and both declined with increasing duration of the disease. Among patients with diabetes for more than 5 years, 11% of adults (18–39 years of age) compared with no adolescents (13–18 years of age) retained insulin secretory capacity. After one year of therapy, intensive glycemic treatment was associated with less of a decline in insulin secretory capacity than standard therapy. Subsequently, the effect of intensive therapy on residual beta cell function was analyzed in 303 of the 855 DCCT patients with diabetes of 1–5 years' duration who had c-peptide responses at baseline.[22] Responders who had been receiving intensive therapy maintained a higher stimulated c-peptide level than responders receiving conventional therapy (57% risk reduction, $p < 0.001$). Maintenance of endogenous insulin secretion was associated with improved metabolic control (Fig. 1), a lower risk of hypoglycemia, and a decreased rate of progression of retinopathy. The mechanism for the protective effect of intensive insulin therapy on islet function is not known. It may be due to a reduction of the glucotoxic effect of hyperglycemia on islet cell function or a slowing of the autoimmune process that leads to islet destruction. Whatever the mechanism, the results in the DCCT strongly support a strategy of intensive glycemic management with insulin from the time of first discovery of type 1 diabetes.

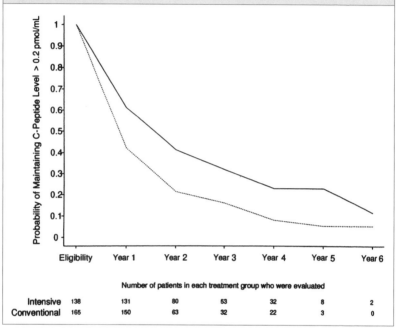

Figure 1. Probability of maintaining c-peptide secretion (stimulated c-peptide level ≥ .20 pmol/ml) with intensive therapy (*solid line*) compared with conventional therapy in the DCCT (*dotted line*) (p<0.001). (From the DCCT Research Group. Ann Intern Med 128:517–523, 1998, with permission.)

Number of patients in each treatment group who were evaluated

	Eligibility	Year 1	Year 2	Year 3	Year 4	Year 5	Year 6
Intensive	138	131	80	53	32	8	2
Conventional	165	150	63	32	22	3	0

In a recently reported phase II trial in 35 patients with type 1 diabetes and residual beta cell function, plasma c-peptide concentrations after glucagon injection were maintained for 10 months in patients treated with an immunomodulatory material, heat shock protein.[14] In the control group, c-peptide levels fell to a significantly greater degree than in the treated group. It was postulated that a shift from a proinflammatory t-helper-1 to an anti-inflammatory t-helper-2 population accounted for the results. Presumably, these promising studies will be followed with large-scale trials to determine whether this therapy can produce long-term maintenance of insulin secretion in type 1 diabetes.

Retinopathy

The DCCT has yielded important longitudinal information about the natural history of microvascular and macrovascular complications in people with type 1 diabetes.[23,30] Long-term information is provided by the ongoing study of DCCT patients in the Epidemiology of Diabetes Interventions and Complications Trial (EDIC).[8,9,18] The study also afforded the best information available about the effect of intensive glycemic management on the natural history of type 1 diabetes and its complications. Because the DCCT led to a major change in guidelines for diabetic care, with a focus on obtaining HbA1c values as close to normal as safely possible, a discussion of the natural history of type 1 diabetes must incorporate major DCCT findings.

At the inception of the DCCT in 1983, the natural history of diabetic retinopathy had been carefully defined from cross-sectional analyses of large numbers of type 1 diabetic patients with varying duration of diabetes. It was clear that retinopathy was a function of duration of the disease and that virtually 100% of people with type 1 diabetes of over 15 years' duration would have some degree of retinopathy. It was also recognized that the disorder can progress in stages: from microaneurysms alone to the addition of hemorrhages, exudates, and microinfarcts[6] to a proliferative process in which friable new vessels may bleed into the retina, macula, and/or vitreous. Laser therapy successfully avoids serious vision loss, if administered properly at the preproliferative or proliferative stage of retinopathy or when vision is threatened by maculopathy.[1,4,10,13] It was recognized that the process proceeded at variable rates and extents in people with type 1 diabetes and that it can be accelerated by hypertension, cigarette smoking, genetic factors, and metabolic control. Some of the evidence related to the effect of glycemic regulation on retinopathy progression was conflicting. Although short-term studies suggested that intensive glycemic management can accelerate preproliferative or proliferative retinopathy, many correlative analyses and animal studies indicated that intensive glycemic management was associated with slower progression.

The design of the DCCT included a group of recently diagnosed type 1 diabetics with disease duration of 1–5 years and no retinopathy to explore the primary prevention of retinopathy (n = 726 patients). A second group had diabetes of up to 15 years' duration and only background retinopathy (n = 715 patients). This group afforded the opportunity to study the effect of glycemic control on existing mild retinopathy—a secondary prevention trial.[17,18,29,30]

The patients were followed for a mean of 6.5 years (range: 3–9 years), and the appearance of retinopathy was assessed by stereophotographs read by masked observers at a central laboratory. Retinopathy was graded according to a precisely defined 25-step scale. Thus, the primary endpoint of the study was objective, unbiased, precise, and clinically significant. Progression of retinopathy in the group assigned to standard therapy was compared with progression in patients treated with intensive glycemic control, and results in the primary and secondary prevention strata were analyzed separately. The median HbA1c in the conventional group was 9.02% and the median HbA1c in the intensively treated group was 7.07% at the final visit, demonstrating a clinically significant difference in long-term glycemic control between the two groups.

Progression of retinopathy was defined as at least a 3-step change from baseline, sustained for at least 6 months. Results in the primary and secondary prevention groups, with conventional or intensive therapy, are shown in Figs. 2A and B. First, it is clear that intensive therapy resulted in retinopathy progression in significantly fewer patients than standard therapy. Second, as predicted from previous cross-sectional studies, 20–30% of patients managed in the conventional way showed significant progression in 5 years, and about 50% progressed after 9 years of type 1 diabetes. Finally, as predicted in earlier studies, there was a transient early worsening in the first year in 13.1% of patients in the secondary prevention group who were assigned to intensive therapy. This finding was significantly less frequent in patients randomized to standard therapy (7.6% of patients; $p < 0.001$). However, no serious visual loss occurred, and the long-term benefits of intensive therapy outweighed the risks of early worsening. Overall, in the primary prevention cohort, intensive therapy reduced the adjusted mean risk for the development of retinopathy by 76% compared with conventional therapy. In the secondary prevention cohort, intensive therapy slowed progression of retinopathy by 54% and the development of proliferative or severe nonproliferative retinopathy by 47%. The relatively flat shapes of the curves over 9 years of study in the intensive group suggested that the beneficial effects of intensive therapy would be long-lasting.

A long-lasting effect of intensive therapy was supported by analyses of retinopathy progression in the two treatment groups 4 years after conclusion of the DCCT.[18] Although the separation in HbA1c between the two groups was no longer present, the group originally randomized into intensive therapy had significantly less progression of retinopathy than the standard group.

The effect of intensive management was to delay the rate of appearance of microaneurysms in the primary prevention cohort compared with the standard management group. However, the risk reduction was only 27%, and at 5 years of therapy approximately 50% of the intensively managed group had one or more microaneurysms compared with close to 70% of patients in the standard group. By life table analysis over 9 years of follow-up, an estimated 7.9% of patients who received intensive treatment would require laser therapy compared with 30% of those with conventional treatment (risk reduction: 59%; $p = 0.001$). Thus, although mild background retinopathy progressed in both groups, serious progression of retinopathy and the need for laser therapy was significantly greater in patients randomized to conventional therapy compared with

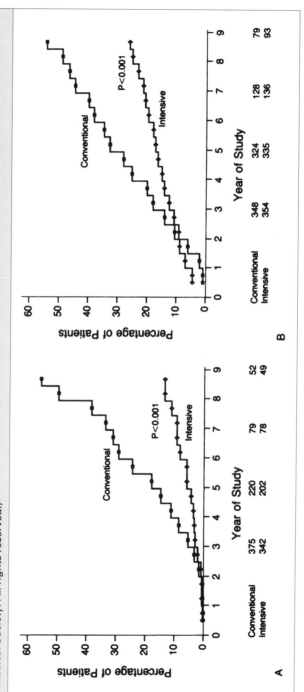

Figure 2. Cumulative incidence of a sustained change in retinopathy in patients with type 1 diabetes receiving intensive or conventional therapy in the DCCT. Results from the primary prevention cohort are shown in panel A, and results from the secondary prevention cohort in panel B. (From the DCCT Research Group. N Eng J Med 329:977–986, 1993, with permission. Copyright© 1993, Massachusetts Medical Society. All rights reserved.)

those in the intensive therapy group. This finding provided strong support for intensive glycemic regulation in type 1 diabetes.

Nephropathy

In the DCCT, renal involvement (nephropathy) was assessed by timed urine collections at baseline and yearly, with calculations of 24-hour urinary albumin excretion and creatinine clearances. Intensive therapy reduced the mean adjusted risk of microalbuminuria, defined as ≥ 40 mg albumin/24 hours, by 34% in the primary prevention group (p = 0.04) and by 43% in the secondary intervention cohort (p = 0.001) (Fig. 3). The risk of albuminuria, defined as ≥ 300 mg/24 hours, was reduced by 86% in the secondary prevention group (p = 0.01).[30] More advanced nephropathy, such as renal failure requiring dialysis, developed in very few patients. The effect of intensive treatment was maintained in various subgroups defined according to age, gender, duration of type 1 diabetes, mean blood pressure, baseline HbA1c, dietary protein intake, or history of cigarette smoking.

Approximately 27% of primary prevention patients assigned to standard therapy had microalbuminuria after 8 years of follow-up compared with only 15% in those in the intensive therapy group. Among secondary prevention patients, approximately 40% assigned to conventional therapy vs. only 25% of these on intensive therapy had microalbuminuria after 9 years in the trial. Thus, although intensive management was effective in delaying progression to microalbuminuria in both primary and secondary prevention cohorts, its appearance was not completely prevented. Analysis during the fourth year after completion of the DCCT in the EDIC Trial showed that the proportion of patients with an increase in urinary albumin excretion continued to be significantly lower in the intensive therapy group.[18] Microalbuminuria has emerged as an important risk marker for renal failure and for cardiovascular events. Additional measures to address these issues are critical and are discussed in other sections of this book.

Neuropathy

Clinically significant neuropathy was defined in the DCCT as an abnormal neurologic examination consistent with peripheral sensorimotor neuropathy plus either abnormal nerve conduction in at least 2 peripheral nerves or abnormal autonomic nerve testing. Among patients in the primary prevention cohort who had no neuropathy at baseline, intensive therapy reduced the appearance of neuropathy at 5 years by 69% (3% vs. 10% in conventional therapy group; p = 0.006). In the secondary prevention group, intensive therapy reduced the appearance of clinical neuropathy at 5 years by 57% (7% vs. 16%, p ≤ 0.001). All three

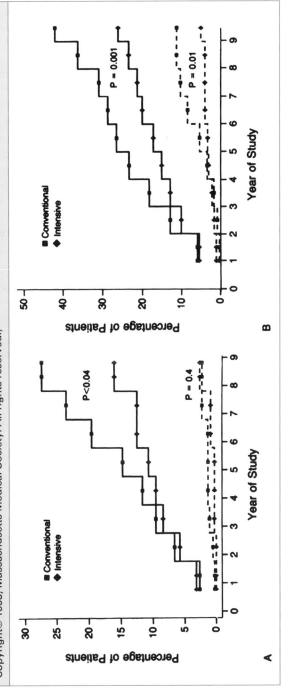

Figure 3. Cumulative incidence of urinary albumin excretion ≥ 300mg/24 hours (*dashed lines*) or ≥ 40 mg/24 hours (*solid lines*) in type 1 patients in the DCCT receiving conventional or intensive therapy. Results in the primary prevention cohort are shown in panel A and from the secondary prevention cohort in panel B. (From the DCCT Research Group N Eng J Med 329:977–986, 1993, with permission. Copyright© 1993, Massachusetts Medical Society. All rights reserved.)

components of neuropathy which were evaluated were reduced by intensive therapy (Fig. 4).[20,21]

Macrovascular Disease

The DCCT cohort was less than 39 years old at entry and was followed for only a mean of 6.5 years. Epidemiologic data had previously suggested that coronary artery disease may become apparent in most type 1 patients only after age 40. Therefore, the macrovascular disease rates in the DCCT were low, and no significant differences between intensive vs. standard management were seen. However, trends suggested a beneficial effect of intensive management to reduce the number of pooled major macrovascular events.[19] An event was defined as death secondary to cardiovascular disease or sudden death, acute myocardial infarction, coronary artery bypass surgery or angioplasty, angina confirmed by angiography, or ischemic changes on noninvasive testing. In addition, major cardiovascular events (fatal or nonfatal stroke) and ma-

Figure 4. Prevalence of abnormal clinical neurologic examinations, abnormal autonomic nerve studies, and abnormal nerve-conduction studies at 5 years in type 1 diabetic patients in the DCCT. Solid bars denote patients receiving intensive therapy; hatched bars indicate patients receiving conventional therapy. (From the DCCT Research Group. N Eng J Med 329:977–986, 1993, with permission. Copyright© 1993, Massachusetts Medical Society. All rights reserved.)

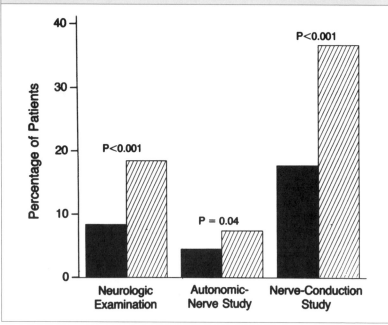

jor peripheral vascular events (amputation, bypass or angioplasty, or claudication with objective evidence) were included.

The number of macrovascular events (40) in the conventionally treated group was greater than that in the intensively treated group (23), but the differences were not statistically significant (p = 0.08). Mean total serum cholesterol and calculated low-density lipoprotein cholesterol were lower in the intensively treated group (p < 0.01), suggesting that long-term benefits may occur.

One of the major goals of the follow-up study of DCCT patients in EDIC is to follow the incidence of macrovascular events in the two treatment groups over a long period. In addition, a variety of cardiovascular risk markers are regularly studied in the two cohorts and will be evaluated as predictors of macrovascular events. In the first report, no significant effect of intensive therapy was seen on carotid artery wall thickness, as an early clinical indicator of arteriosclerosis.[9] These studies were done 1–2 years after completion of the DCCT in the EDIC study and will be repeated at intervals during a planned 10-year follow-up of DCCT patients to see whether long-term changes will be seen.

Diabetic nephropathy has a major impact on cardiovascular disease in type 1 diabetes.[33] In a long-term study of 5148 type 1 diabetics diagnosed in Finland between 1965 and 1979, Tuomilehto et al. found that the cumulative incidence of cardiovascular disease was 43% in type 1 diabetic patients with nephropathy compared with 7% in those without nephropathy. The cumulative incidence of coronary heart disease, stroke, and all cardiovascular disease in both groups increased as a function of the duration of type of diabetes. It also increased as a function of age of the patients and duration of nephropathy.

These figures are expected to improve in future years with intensive therapy for the hyperglycemia, hypertension, microalbuminuria, and lipid/lipoprotein alterations that characterize diabetic nephropathy.

Pregnancy

Before the DCCT, it had been conclusively demonstrated that intensive glycemic management before and during pregnancy markedly improved fetal mortality and morbidity.[2] Accordingly, whenever a patient was actively pursuing pregnancy during the trial (or when pregnancy was diagnosed), she was immediately placed on intensive management, whether initially randomized into the conventional or intensive management group.

A total of 180 women in the DCCT completed 270 pregnancies, with 191 total live births.[27] HbA1c values differed at conception (intensive, 7.4%; conventional, 8.1%), but were similar in both groups during pregnancy (6.6%). There were no significant differences in outcome between the women with conventional treatment who initiated intensive therapy before conception and those who began it after conception. Intensive therapy was associated with rates of spontaneous abortion and congenital malformations similar to those in the nondiabetic population. Thus, the DCCT findings supported recommendations that intensive management should be initiated in all women with type 1 diabetes who are planning pregnancy or who are pregnant.

The DCCT afforded an opportunity to explore the effect of pregnancy in type 1 diabetes on progression of retinopathy and albuminuria.[24] Furthermore, the effect of prior randomization into the conventional or intensive treatment group was assessed. In accord with other studies, there was a transient increase in the risk of progression of retinopathy during pregnancy in the DCCT. In the intensive group, there was a 1.63-fold greater risk of worsening of retinopathy from before to during pregnancy compared with nonpregnant women. This risk was 2.48-fold greater in the conventional group compared with nonpregnant women. The odds ratio peaked during the second trimester and persisted as long as 12 months after pregnancy. Small changes in albumin excretion rates were within the normal range in most subjects. It is significant, however, that the long-term risk of progression of retinopathy and albumin excretion, as assessed at the end of the DCCT, was not affected by pregnancy.[24]

In view of the transient increase in the risk of retinopathy progression during pregnancy in type 1 diabetes, increased ophthalmologic surveillance is indicated.

Weight

In the DCCT, intensively treated patients gained an average of 4.75 kg more than conventionally treated patients ($p < 0.0001$).[26,31] This finding represented an excessive increase in BMI of 1.5 kg/m^2 in men and 1.8 kg/m^2 in women. Weight gain was most rapid in the first year of therapy. By year 9 of the study, BMIs had increased >5 kg/m^2 in 35% of women and 28% of men, whereas comparable figures in the conventionally treated women and men were approximately 13% and 4%.

Waist-to-hip ratio did not differ between treatment groups. However, intensively treated DCCT subjects who were in the highest quartile of weight gain had increased waist-hip ratios and BMIs, associated with a slightly higher blood pressure and a relatively atherogenic lipid profile. These patients may be predisposed to the insulin resistance syndrome, and their tendency for abdominal obesity may have been exposed by intensive insulin therapy. Long-term follow-up of these patients in EDIC will be of great interest.

Among patients without major weight gain, those on intensive therapy had a greater fat-free mass with no difference in adiposity. Although the benefits of intensive management on microvascular complications in type 1 diabetes are clear, improved understanding of the causes of weight gain and methods to control it are needed.

Hypoglycemia

The major adverse event in the DCCT was a threefold increase in the incidence of severe hypoglycemia in the intensively treated group.[15,25] Severe hypoglycemia was defined as an episode with symptoms consistent with hypoglycemia, in which the patient required the assistance of another person and which was associated with a blood glucose level <50 mg/dl or prompt recovery after oral carbohydrate, glucagon, or IV glucose. A total of 65% of patients in the intensive group had at least one episode of severe hypoglycemia vs. 35% of patients in the conventional therapy group. Overall rates were 61.2 per 100 years in the intensive group and 18.7 per 100 years in the conventional group. A history of severe hypoglycemia in the past was the best predictor.

Subgroup analyses showed that males, adolescents, and patients with no residual c-peptide secretion had a particularly high rate of severe hypoglycemia in both treatment groups. Intensive treatment was also associated with an increased risk of multiple episodes of severe hypoglycemia within the same patient. Approximately 25–30% of intensively treated patients vs. 5–11% of the conventional group had severe hypoglycemia each year, and about 10–12% vs. 3–5% resulted in a coma or seizure respectively in the two treatment groups. No changes in neuropsychological function were noted.[20]

The DCCT investigators concluded that intensive management of type 1 diabetes, with a goal of normal or near-normal levels of glycemia, is associated with an increased risk of severe hypoglycemia. Individualization of therapeutic goals and methods was encouraged. In particular, future development of intensive treatment methods that afford the benefits of improved glucose control with reduced risks of hypoglycemia was advocated.

Hypoglycemia unawareness is frequently seen in type 1 diabetics after prolonged periods of intensive glucose regulation and recurrent hypoglycemic attacks.[12] This issue has received extensive study.[7] It has been postulated that in hypoglycemia-aware type 1 patients, beta-adrenergic sensitivity is increased to compensate for impaired catecholamine response. With repeated episodes of hypoglycemia, this increased sensitivity is lost. The end result is hypoglycemia unawareness with reduced catecholamine response and reduced beta-adrenergic sensitivity. Recent studies have shown that this sensitivity may be restored in type 1 diabetes by avoiding hypoglycemia with less stringent blood glucose control.[11] Thus, in patients with hypoglycemia unawareness, it is appropriate to modify the stringent HbA1c and plasma glucose control goals to avoid recurrent hypoglycemia and hypoglycemic unawareness.

Key Points: Type 1 Diabetes

- Autoimmune destruction of the pancreatic beta cells is the major cause of type 1 diabetes.
- Type 1 diabetes is a genetically determined disorder; the genes responsible are within the major histocompatibility complex located on chromosome 6.
- Evidence of residual insulin secretion is present in 45% of adults (ages 18–39 years) within 5 years after the onset of type 1 diabetes, and 11% retain some secretory capacity after 5 years of type 1 diabetes.
- Intensive glycemic therapy may result in the maintenance of some insulin secretory capacity. This is associated with improved metabolic control, less hypoglycemia, and slower progression of retinopathy than in intensively managed patients with no insulin secretory capacity.
- Intensive team management of type 1 diabetic patients with no retinopathy, with a therapeutic goal of normoglycemia, results in a 76% reduction in the risk for the development of clinically significant retinopathy compared with conventional management.
- A beneficial effect on retinopathy progression is maintained for at least 4 years after a prolonged period (mean: 6.5 years) of intensive management.
- Significant effects of intensive management include a decrease in urinary albumin excretion (an index of nephropathy) and a reduction in clinical evidence of peripheral sensory and autonomic neuropathy.
- Favorable trends occur in macrovascular endpoints with intensive management of type 1 diabetes.
- Intensive management improves outcomes of pregnancy in type 1 diabetes.
- Although transient increases in retinopathy progression occur during pregnancy and in some patients with intensive management, the long-term risk of progression of retinopathy is not affected.
- Increased ophthalmologic surveillance during pregnancy in type 1 diabetes is indicated.
- The two main adverse effects of intensive management of type 1 diabetes are weight gain and an increased incidence of severe hypoglycemia.
- Intensive treatment methods of type 1 diabetes have been under study since the completion of the DCCT with goals of decreasing the risks of excessive weight gain and severe hypoglycemia.

Key Points (*Continued*)

⇨ Long-term follow-up of the DCCT cohort in the EDIC Trial will provide valuable natural history data and information on the effects of a defined period of intensive glycemic management on microvascular and macrovascular complications.

References

1. American Diabetes Association: Diabetic retinopathy. Diabetes Care 25:S90–S93, 2002.
2. American Diabetes Association: Preconception care of women with diabetes. Diabetes Care 25:S82–S84, 2002.
3. American Diabetes Association: Prevention of type 1 diabetes. Diabetes Care 25:S131, 2002.
4. American Diabetes Association: Standards of medical care for patients with diabetes mellitus. Diabetes Care 25:S33–S49, 2002.
5. Atkinson MA, Maclaren NK: The pathogenesis of insulin-dependent diabetes mellitus. N Eng J Med 331:1428–1436, 1994.
6. Boeri D, Maiello M, Lorenzi M: Increased prevalence of microthromboses in retinal capillaries of diabetic individuals. Diabetes 50:1432–1439, 2001.
7. Cryer PE: Banting Lecture. Hypoglycemia: the limiting factor in the management of IDDM. Diabetes 43:1378–1389, 1994.
8. Epidemiology of Diabetes Interventions and Complications (EDIC) Research Group: Design, implementation, and preliminary results of a long-term follow-up of the Diabetes Control and Complications Trial cohort. Diabetes Care 22:99–111, 1999.
9. Epidemiology of Diabetes Interventions and Complications (EDIC) Research Group: Effect of intensive diabetes treatment on carotid artery wall thickness in the epidemiology of diabetes interventions and complications. Diabetes 48:383–390, 1999.
10. Ferris FL III, Davis MD, Aiello LM: Treatment of diabetic retinopathy. N Engl J Med 341:667–678, 1999.
11. Fritsche A, Stefan N, Haring H, et al: Avoidance of hypoglycemia restores hypoglycemia awareness by increasing β-adrenergic sensitivity in type 1 diabetes. Ann Intern Med 134:729–736, 2001.
12. Gerich JE, Mokan M. Beneman T, et al: Hypoglycemia unawareness. Endocr Rev. 12:356–371, 1991.
13. Klein R: Diabetic retinopathy: An end of the century perspective. Eye 13:133–135, 1999.
14. Raz I, Elias, D, Avron A, et al: β-cell function in new-onset type 1 diabetes and immunomodulation with a heat-shock protein peptide (DiaPep277): A randomised, double-blind, phase II trial. Lancet 358:1749–1753, 2001.
15. Diabetes Control and Complications Trial Research Group: Adverse events and their association with treatment regimens in the diabetes control and complications trial. Diabetes Care 18:1145–1427, 1995.
16. Diabetes Control and Complications Trial Research Group: Clustering of long-term complications in families with diabetes in the diabetes control and complications trial. Diabetes 46:1829–1839, 1997.
17. Diabetes Control and Complications Trial Research Group: Progression of retinopathy

with intensive versus conventional treatment in the diabetes control and complications trial. Ophthalmology 102:647–661, 1995.

18. Diabetes Control and Complications Trial/Epidemiology of Diabetes Interventions and Complications Research Group. Retinopathy and Nephropathy in patients with type 1 diabetes four years after a trial of intensive therapy. N Engl J Med 342:381–389, 2000.

19. Diabetes Control and Complications Trial (DCCT) Research Group: Effect of intensive diabetes management on macrovascular events and risk factors in the diabetes control and complications trial. Am J. Cardiol 75:894–903, 1995.

20. Diabetes Control and Complications Trial Research Group: Effects of intensive diabetes therapy on neuropsychological function in adults in the Diabetes Control and Complications Trial. Ann Intern Med 124:379–388, 1996.

21. Diabetes Control and Complications Trial Research Group: The effect of intensive diabetes therapy on the development and progression of neuropathy. Ann Intern Med 122:561–568, 1995.

22. Diabetes Control and Complications Trial Research Group: Effect of intensive therapy on residual β-cell function in patients with type 1 diabetes in the diabetes control and complications trial. Ann Intern Med 128:517–523, 1998.

23. Diabetes Control and Complications Trial Research Group: Effect of intensive diabetes treatment on the development and progression of long-term complications in adolescents with insulin-dependent diabetes mellitus: Diabetes Control and Complications Trial. J Pediatrics 125:177–188, 1994.

24. Diabetes Control and Complications Trial Research Group: Effect of pregnancy on microvascular complications in the Diabetes Control and Complications Trial. Diabetes Care 23:1084–1091, 2000.

25. Diabetes Control and Complications Trial Research Group: Hypoglycemia in the Diabetes Control and Complications Trial. Diabetes 46:271–286, 1997.

26. Diabetes Control and Complications Trial Research Group: Influence of intensive diabetes treatment on body weight and composition of adults with type 1 diabetes in the Diabetes Control and Complications Trial. Diabetes Care 24:1711–1721, 2001.

27. Diabetes Control and Complications Trial Research Group: Pregnancy outcomes in the Diabetes Control and Complications Trial. Am J Obstet Gynecol 174:1343–1353, 1996.

28. Diabetes Control and Complications Trial Research Group: The effect of intensive diabetes therapy on measures of autonomic nervous system function in the Diabetes Control and Complications Trial (DCCT). Diabetologia 41:416–423, 1998.

29. Diabetes Control and Complications Trial Research Group: The effect of intensive diabetes treatment on the progression of diabetic retinopathy in insulin-dependent diabetes mellitus. Arch Ophthalmol 113:36–51, 1995.

30. Diabetes Control and Complications Trial Research Group: The effect of intensive treatment of diabetes on the development and progression of long-term complications in insulin-dependent diabetes mellitus. N Engl J Med 329:977–986, 1993.

31. DCCT Research Group: Weight gain associated with intensive therapy in the diabetes control and complications trial. Diabetes Care 11:567–573, 1988.

32. Expert Committee on the Diagnosis and Classification of Diabetes Mellitus: Report of the expert committee on the diagnosis and classification of diabetes mellitus. Diabetes Care 20:1183–1197,1997.

33. Tuomilehto J, Borch-Johnson K, Molarius A, et al: Incidence of cardiovascular disease in type 1 (insulin-dependent) diabetic subjects with and without diabetic nephropathy in Finland. Diabetologia 41:784–790, 1998.

Guidelines for Diabetes Care

chapter

4

Diabetes Self-Management Education

Diabetes self-management education (DSME) is critical to successful care for all people with type 1 and type 2 diabetes. National standards for DSME are regularly updated by the American Diabetes Association and are reviewed and approved by key organizations with involvement in diabetes care.

The 10 national standards for DSME are comprehensive and fully described in the Clinical Practice Recommendations of the American Diabetes Association.[18] The ADA has a recognition program for hospitals, clinics, and other health care sites that develop programs in accord with these guidelines. Reimbursement for DSME from Medicare is linked to ADA recognition. The 10 standards can be summarized as follows:

1. Documentation of organizational structure, mission and goals, and recognition of quality DSME as an integral component of diabetes care.
2. Definition of target population, its educational needs, and necessary resources.
3. Oversight by a representative advisory body, including planning, ongoing review of outcomes, and consideration of community concerns.
4. Designation of a qualified coordinator.
5. Interaction of the patient with diabetes with a multifaceted education instructional team, which should include at least a registered dietician and a registered nurse who are certified diabetes educators (or eligible to become a CDE).
6. Regular continuing education for the instructors.
7. A written curriculum, with criteria for successful learning outcomes.
8. Individualized assessment, development of an educational plan, and reassessment of participants.
9. Documentation of step 8 in a confidential education record.
10. Development of a continuous quality improvement process.

Medical Nutrition and Exercise Therapy

An individualized meal plan is essential to aid in achieving the goals of therapy. It should include a nutrition assessment and plan with specific identified goals.[5] This plan should be initiated and reinforced by a registered dietician who optimally is a certified diabetes educator. Because the approaches to nutrition therapy differ in patients with type 1 and type 2 diabetes, further discussion is included in relevant chapters.

As part of nutrition and/or overall diabetes education, an exercise program is essential.[2] Evaluation of the patient before exercise and an individualized prescription geared to the type of diabetes, presence of complications, drug therapy, and goals for weight are necessary. Specific examples for type 1 and type 2 diabetic patients are included in later chapters.

Clinical Assessments

A group of clinical assessments is defined for optimal diabetes care. Specific goals of therapy are linked to these assessments and, in general, are based on evidence from randomized collaborative therapeutic trials.[9] These assessments are described below, with brief reviews of the evidence in support of their use.

Glucose

Experiences from the DCCT are examples of the evidence-based background that supports intensive management of type 1 diabetes. This landmark study demonstrated that intensive therapy aimed at achieving glycemic control as close to normal as possible reduced the development and progression of retinopathy, albuminuria, and neuropathy compared with conventional therapy. The findings of this randomized trial are extended and supported by epidemiologic studies of the level of glycemic exposure before and during the DCCT with the risk of progression of the primary endpoint, retinopathy.

Total glycemic exposure emerged as the dominant factor defining the risk of development and progression of retinopathy in the DCCT.[20] The shorter the duration of type 1 diabetes at entry into the trial and the lower the baseline HbA1c value, the greater the benefits of intensive therapy. Within each treatment group. the mean HbA1c during the trial was the dominant predictor of retinopathy progression (Fig. 1)

A second important finding in the DCCT was that there was no level of glycemia below which the risks of retinopathy progression were eliminated. However, the risk over time differed in the two treatment groups: it increased in the conventional group and remained relatively constant in the intensive group (Fig. 2) Total glycemic exposure was the dominant fac-

Figure 1. The rate per 100 patient years of sustained retinopathy progression within quintiles of updated mean HbA1c (percentage) during the study and within quintiles of the distribution of time of follow-up during the study (years). *A,* Conventional treatment group. *B,* Intensive treatment group. (From the DCCT Research Group. Diabetes 44:968–983, 1995, with permission.)

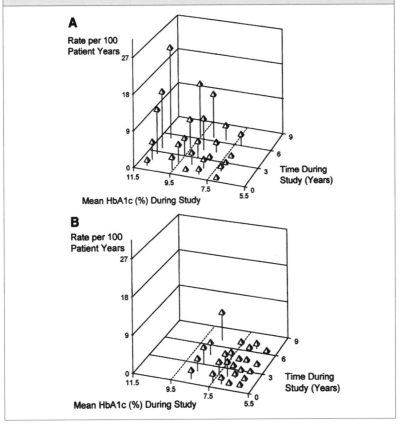

tor associated with the risk of retinopathy progression. Similar results were seen when progression of albuminuria or neuropathy was examined.

Further analyses indicated that there was no glycemic threshold below which no further reduction in risk was seen.[19] The risks of retinopathy progression and of developing microalbuminuria and neuropathy were continuous and nonlinear over the entire range of HbA1c values in the study. Proportional reductions in HbA1c were accompanied by proportional reduction in the risks of complications.

The absolute risks of sustained retinopathy progression over the HbA1c range observed in the DCCT are shown in Fig. 2. It is apparent that the risks increase in a curvilinear fashion in the conventional group,

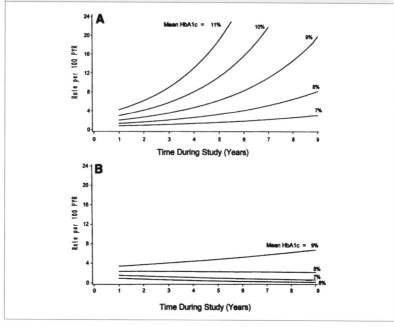

Figure 2. Absolute risk of sustained retinopathy as a function of the updated mean HbA1c (percentage) during the study and the time of follow-up during the study (years). A, Conventional treatment group. B, Intensive treatment group. (From the DCCT Research Group. Diabetes 44:968–983, 1995, with permission.)

that there is no apparent threshold, and that any degree of lowering of HbA1c is associated with a decreased risk for these microvascular endpoints, especially in patients with HbA1c levels ≥8%.

Experiences in the United Kingdom Prospective Diabetes Study (UKPDS) in newly diagnosed type 2 diabetics have supported the DCCT findings on glycemic regulation and retinopathy progression in type 1 diabetes. The UKPDS is considered in more detail in a future chapter.

These data form the primary basis for the current recommendations by the American Diabetes Association for glycemic management of diabetes.[9] The guidelines are given in Table 1.

These guidelines may be modified in patients with comorbid diseases, very young or older adults, and others with unusual conditions (i.e., recurrent hypoglycemia). HbA1c should be measured quarterly if therapeutic goals are not met and at least twice yearly in all diabetic patients.

Lipids/Lipoproteins

Guidelines for optimal control of plasma lipid or lipoproteins in diabetes mellitus are based on the recognition that both type 1 and type 2

TABLE 1.	Glycemic Control Guidelines: Diabetes Mellitus		
	Normal	Goal (mg/dl)	Action
Whole blood values*			
Average preprandial glucose	<100	80–120	<80 >140
Average bedtime glucose	<110	100–140	<100 >160
Plasma values†			
Average preprandial glucose	<110	90–130	<90 >150
Average bedtime glucose	<120	110–150	<110 >180
HbA1c	<6%	<7%	>8%

*Capillary blood glucose
†Venous plasma glucose

diabetic patients have disordered lipid metabolism. In type 1 diabetes, elevations of triglycerides, low HDL-cholesterol and elevation of LDL cholesterol are particularly dependent on poor glycemic control and tend to return to normal with intensive insulin therapy.[17] An atherogenic lipoprotein profile usually accompanies diabetic nephropathy. People with type 1 diabetes have a shortened lifespan that is due primarily either to renal insufficiency or to cardiovascular events—and, often a combination of both. Thus, strict guidelines for lipoprotein control apply to people with type 1 diabetes. In type 2 diabetes, dyslipidemia is often characterized by low plasma HDL-C, high plasma triglyceride levels, and a population of small, dense LDL particles, which are particularly atherogenic. Cardiovascular disease is the major cause of death in type 2 diabetes, and dyslipidemia is probably a major contributor.

In type 2 diabetes (in contrast to type 1 diabetes), abundant evidence from prospective randomized trials shows that intensive management of lipids and lipoproteins is indicated to reduce the risk for cardiovascular events. This subject is covered in detail in future chapters. There is now substantial agreement between the American Diabetes Association[6] and the National Cholesterol Education Program[15] regarding guidelines for therapy of lipids and lipoproteins in adults with diabetes mellitus. The goals of therapy are as follows:

TABLE 2.	Guidelines for Plasma Levels of Lipids/Lipoproteins After an Overnight Fast
Cholesterol:	<200mg/dl
LDL cholesterol:	< 100mg/dl
HDL cholesterol:	>45mg/dl (men)
	>55mg/dl (women)
Triglycerides:	<150mg/dl

Lipid profiles should be measured yearly in people with diabetes, and more frequently when changes in dietary or drug management are made. These guidelines can be viewed from another perspective (Table 3).

TABLE 3. Category of Risk Based on Lipid/ Lipoprotein Levels in Adults With Diabetes			
Risk	LDL Cholesterol*	LDL Cholesterol*	Triglyceride*
High	≥130	< 35	≥400
Borderline	100–129	35–45	200–399
Low	<100	>45	<200

*mg/dl. For women, raise HDL cholesterol by 10 mg/dl.

Dilated Eye Examination

The presence of diabetic retinopathy is strongly related to the duration of diabetes. After 20 years of diabetes, virtually all type 1 and 60–70% of type 2 diabetics have evidence of retinopathy. In type 2 diabetes, duration may be difficult to determine accurately, and approximately 20% may have retinopathy at the time of first recognition of diabetes. In the first 5 years of type 1 diabetes, vision-threatening retinopathy is rarely seen. Factors that affect progression or retinopathy are glycemic control, hypertension, and pregnancy. There is an association between plasma lipid levels and hard exudates, which usually are found in the macular region. Regular dilated eye examinations are necessary to diagnose retinal or macular changes that may be amenable to laser photocoagulation. The efficacy and safety of this procedure has been scientifically demonstrated in two major National Institutes of Health sponsored trials: the Diabetic Retinopathy Study[21,22,23] and the Early Treatment Diabetic Retinopathy Study (ETDRS).[24,25,26,27]

The guidelines for dilated eye examinations by an ophthalmologist or an optometrist who is experienced in the diagnosis of diabetic retinopathy are shown in Table 4.[4]

TABLE 4. Ophthalmologic Examination Schedule in People With Diabetes		
Patient Group‡	First Examination	Minimum Follow-up*
1. 29 years or younger	Within 3–5 years of diagnosis†	Yearly
2. 30 years and older	At time of diagnosis	Yearly
pregnancy and diabetes	Before conception and in first trimester	Depends on results (1st trimester)

*Abnormal findings: increase frequency.
†Age 10 years or older; clinical judgment for <10 years.
‡Age delineation reflects system used in the Wisconsin Epidemiologic Study of Diabetic Retinopathy (WESDR).[16] The majority of patients in group 1 have type 1 diabetes; in group 2, the majority have type 2 diabetes.

Blood Pressure

Hypertension is more prevalent in people with diabetes than in age- and gender-matched nondiabetics. In type 1 diabetes, an elevation of blood pressure is usually seen concomitant with the development of microalbuminuria and is present in 18–33% of people with type 1 diabetes.[14,16] Hypertension is at least twice as prevalent in people with type 2 diabetes than in nondiabetic individuals and is a frequent finding in the metabolic syndrome. African Americans have a very high prevalence of hypertension. Elevated blood pressure is a major contributor to cardiovascular mortality and morbidity, renal failure, retinopathy progression, strokes, peripheral vascular disease, and amputations in diabetic subjects.

In recent years, there has been an explosion of information from large scale collaborative clinical trials that aggressive treatment of elevated blood pressure in people with diabetes has major benefits in preserving renal function and reducing the incidence of cardiovascular events. These studies are reviewed in detail in another chapter.

Presently, the consensus between the American Diabetes Association[10] and the National Kidney Foundation[11] is that the goal for therapy in adults with diabetes is to achieve a blood pressure < 130/80 mmHg. The ADA suggests some modification of these goals in patients with isolated systolic hypertension (Table 5)

Urinary Albumin

It has become clear in recent years that a small excess of albumin in the urine (microalbuminuria) is a predictor of progressive renal disease in people with type 1 diabetes and a risk marker for cardiovascular death in type 2 diabetes. Furthermore, large-scale collaborative trials have indicated that angiotensin-converting enzyme inhibitors (ACE-1) slow the progression of renal insufficiency in types 1 and 2 diabetes and decrease cardiovascular events in type 2 diabetic patients.[3] Angiotensin receptor blockers (ARBs) delay progression of renal failure in type 2 diabetics with nephropathy. This important area is considered in more detail in another chapter.

TABLE 5. Blood Pressure Goals in Diabetes Mellitus		
Hypertension	**B.P. Patient mm/Hg**	**B.P. Goal**
Systolic and diastolic	>130/80	<130/80
Isolated systolic	≥180	<160*
	160–179	140–159*
*If tolerated, further reduction to 140 mmHg is appropriate.		

In view of these facts, screening for urinary albumin is recommended in all people with diabetes. Testing should be done after 5 years duration of type 1 diabetes and at the time of diagnosis in type 2 diabetes. A 24-hour collection, a timed urine collection, or a spot collection may be obtained. The usual urine dipstick is not sensitive enough to detect microalbuminuria. Critical values of urinary albumin excretion are shown in Table 6.

Foot Examination

Foot ulcers and amputations are a major cause of morbidity and increased costs for people with diabetes. Studies have shown that identification of people at risk for ulcers and/or amputation is critical and that preventive therapy, particularly for those at risk, is often effective. Risk for ulcer or amputation is increased in people who have had diabetes ≥10 years, are male, have poor glucose control, or have cardiovascular, renal, or retinal complications. Amputation incidence is rising in many medical centers. Risk factors that can be identified on examination include peripheral neuropathy with decreased sensation, altered foot biomechanics with neuropathy (callus or bony deformity), and decreased posterior tibial or pedal pulses.

Care guidelines, therefore, include an annual foot examination for all patients with diabetes and at every visit for those with peripheral neuropathy.[7] Education about risk and prevention of foot problems is indicated, and specific issues of care (including referral) are considered in another chapter.

Smoking Assessment

Epidemiologic studies show a clear relationship between cigarette smoking and health risks. In diabetics, cigarette smoking magnifies the already high risk for cardiovascular disease and also accelerates microvascular disease, particularly of the retina. Nevertheless, approximately 20% of people with diabetes in the U.S. continue to smoke cig-

TABLE 6.	Critical Values of Urinary Albumin Excretion		
Category	24-hr Collection (mg/24 hrs)	Timed Collection (μg/min)	Spot Collection (μg/mg Cr.)
Normal	<30	<20	<30
Microalbuminuria	30–299	20–199	30–299
Clinical albuminuria	≥300	≥200	≥300

Because of variability in urinary albumin excretion, two of three specimens collected within a 3- to 6-month period should be abnormal before considering a patient to have crossed one of these diagnostic thresholds. Exercise within 24 hr, infection, fever, congestive heart failure, marked hyperglycemia, marked hypertension, pyuria, and hematuria may elevate urinary albumin excretion over baseline values.

arettes, and attention to this issue is important in overall care for people with diabetes.[8] Specific recommendations about diabetes and smoking are given in Table 7.[8]

Aspirin Therapy

Aspirin therapy is indicated in some but not all patients with type 1 diabetes.[1,12,13] Most of the controlled trial data has been obtained in subjects with type 2 diabetes who have already had a cardiovascular event or who are at high risk for an event because of a family history of coronary heart disease, cigarette smoking, hypertension, overweight, albuminuria, altered lipid profile (cholesterol >200 mg/dl; LDL-C >100 mg/dl; HDL-C < 45 mg/dl in men or < 55 mg/dl in women), or age >30 years.

The consensus is that type 1 diabetics age 30 or over, who have had a vascular event or one or more cardiovascular risk factors should receive aspirin therapy. Low doses (81–325 mg/day) of enteric-coated aspirin are recommended to provide adequate blockade of thromboxane release and to afford some protection against gastrointestinal tract irritation. Many diabetic patients have nephropathy and/or hypertension, and aspirin therapy is clearly indicated in this group if hypertension is controlled. On the other hand, because of the lack of controlled information in type 1 patients under age 30 and because of the risk of Reye's syndrome, aspirin therapy should not be recommended under the age of 21 years.

Clopidogrel is also an effective antiplatelet agent but has been studied primarily in nondiabetics. It can be used as a substitute for aspirin, particularly in the case of aspirin allergy.

TABLE 7. Recommendations Regarding Diabetes and Smoking
Assessment of smoking status and history
• Obtain systematic documentation of a history of tobacco use.
Counseling on smoking prevention and cessation
• Advise people with diabetes not to initiate smoking. Consistently repeat the advice to prevent smoking and other tobacco use among children and adolescents with diabetes under age 21 years.
• Provide cessation counseling in smokers as a routine component of diabetes care. Urge every smoker to quit in a clear, strong, and personalized manner that describes the added risks of smoking and diabetes.
• Ask every person with diabetes who is a smoker if he or she is willing to quit. Initiate a motivational discussion regarding the need to stop using tobacco, the risks of continued use, and encouragement to quit as well as support when ready.
• Offer pharmacologic supplements as appropriate.
• Arrange follow-up procedures designed to assess and promote quitting status for all people with diabetes who are smokers.

TABLE 8. Summary of Guidelines for Diabetes Care		
Assessment	**Frequency**	**Goal**
Diabetic education	Based on assessment	Understanding diabetes
Medical nutrition therapy	Based on assessment	Optimal weight
HbA1c	Twice yearly*	<7%
Cholesterol	Yearly*	<200 mg/dl
LDL-C	Yearly*	<100 mg/dl
HDL-C	Yearly*	>45 mg/dl(M) >55 mg/dl(F)
Triglyceride	Yearly*	<150 mg/dl
Dilated eye exam	Yearly†	Prevent progression
Blood pressure	Each visit	<130/80 mmHg
Urinary albumin	Yearly*†	<30 mg/24 hr.
Foot exam	Each Visit	Prevent amputation
Smoking assessment	Yearly	Prevent CV events
Aspirin therapy‡	Daily	Prevent CV events

CV = cardiovascular.
*Quarterly if on drug therapy, until at goal.
†Except type 1 diabetes <10 yrs of age or within 5 years of diagnosis.
‡Over age 30: high cardiovascular risk.

Key Points: Aspirin Therapy

↪ Aspirin therapy (81–325 mg of enteric-coated aspirin/day) should be given to type 1 diabetic patients over age 30 who have had a cardiovascular event or are at high risk for cardiovascular events.

↪ Many of these type 1 diabetic patients have nephropathy and/or hypertension.

↪ Clopidogrel may be used as a substitute in patients with aspirin allergy.

↪ Table 8 summarizes guidelines for care.

References

1. American Diabetes Association: Aspirin therapy in diabetes. Diabetes Care 25:S78–S79, 2002.
2. American Diabetes Association: Diabetes mellitus and exercise. Diabetes Care 25:S64–S68, 2002.
3. American Diabetes Association: Diabetic nephropathy. Diabetes Care 25:S85–S89, 2002.
4. American Diabetes Association: Diabetic retinopathy. Diabetes Care 25:S90–S93, 2002.
5. American Diabetes Association: Evidence-based nutrition principles and recommendations for the treatment and prevention of diabetes and related complications. Diabetes Care 25:S50–S60, 2002.

6. American Diabetes Association: Management of dyslipidemia in adults with diabetes. Diabetes Care 25:S74–S77, 2002.
7. American Diabetes Association: Preventive foot care in people with diabetes. Diabetes Care 25:S69–S70, 2002.
8. American Diabetes Association: Smoking and diabetes. Diabetes Care 25:S80–S81, 2002.
9. American Diabetes Association: Standards of medical care for patients with diabetes mellitus. Diabetes Care 25:S33–S49, 2002.
10. American Diabetes Association: Treatment of hypertension in adults with diabetes. Diabetes Care 25:S71–S73, 2002.
11. Bakris GL, Williams M, Dworkin L, et al: Special Report: Preserving renal function in adults with hypertension and diabetes: A consensus approach. Am J Kidney Dis 36:646–661, 2000.
12. Colwell JA: Aspirin therapy in diabetes [position statement]. Diabetes Care 20:1772–1773, 1997.
13. Colwell JA. Aspirin therapy in diabetes [Technical Review]. Diabetes Care, 20:1767–1771, 1997.
14. Epidemiology of Diabetes Interventions and Complications (EDIC) Research Group: Design, implementation, and preliminary results of a long-term follow-up of the Diabetes Control and Complications Trial cohort . Diabetes Care 22:99–111, 1999.
15. Executive Summary of the Third Report of the National Cholesterol Education Program (NCEP) Expert Panel on Detection, Evaluation, and Treatment of High Blood Cholesterol in Adults (Adult Treatment Panel III). JAMA 285:2486–2497, 2001.
16. Klein R, Klein BEK, Moss SE, et al: The 10-year incidence of renal insufficiency in people with Type 1 diabetes. Diabetes Care 22:743–751, 1999.
17. Lopes-Virella MF, Wohltmann HJ, Mayfield RK, et al: Effect of metabolic control on lipid, lipoprotein, and apolipoprotein levels in 55 insulin-dependent diabetic patients: A longitudinal study. Diabetes 32:20–25, 1983.
18. Mensing C, Boucher J, Cypress, M, et al: National standards for diabetes self-management education. Diabetes Care 25:S140–S147, 2002.
19. The Diabetes Control and Complications Trial Research Group: Perspectives in diabetes: The absence of a glycemic threshold for the development of long-term complications: The perspective of the Diabetes Control and Complications Trial. Diabetes 45:1289–1298, 1996.
20. The Diabetes Control and Complications Trial Research Group: The relationship of glycemic exposure (HbA1c) to the risk of development and progression of retinopathy in the Diabetes Control and Complications Trial. Diabetes 44:968–983, 1995.
21. The Diabetic Retinopathy Study Research Group. Preliminary report on effects of photocoagulation therapy. Am J Ophthalmol 81:383–396, 1976.
22. The Diabetic Retinopathy Study Research Group. Photocoagulation treatment of proliferative diabetic retinopathy. Clinical application of Diabetic Retinopathy Study (DRS) findings, DRS Report Number 8. Ophthalmology 88:583–600, 1981.
23. The Diabetic Retinopathy Study Research Group: Photocoagulation treatment of proliferative diabetic retinopathy: The second report of Diabetic Retinopathy Study findings. Ophthalmology 85:82–105, 1978.
24. The Early Treatment Diabetic Retinopathy Study Research Group: Early photocoagulation for diabetic retinopathy: ETDRS report no. 9. Ophthalmology 98:766–785, 1991.
25. The Early Treatment Diabetic Retinopathy Study Research Group. Photocoagulation for diabetic macular edema. Early Treatment Diabetic Retinopathy Study Report Number 1. Arch Ophthalmol 103:1796–1806, 1985.

26. The Early Treatment Diabetic Retinopathy Study Research Group: Techniques for scatter and local photocoagulation treatment of diabetic retinopathy: early Treatment Diabetic Retinopathy Study Report No. 3. Int Ophthalmol Clin 27:254–264, 1987.

27. The Early Treatment Diabetic Retinopathy Study Research Group. Treatment techniques and clinical guidelines for photocoagulation of diabetic macular edema. Early Treatment Diabetic Retinopathy Study Report Number 2. Ophthalmology 94:761–774, 1987.

Intensive Management of Type 1 Diabetes

chapter
5

Conceptual Framework

Type 1 diabetes is characterized by insulin deficiency. Although small amounts of insulin reserve may be present in the first few years after diagnosis, insulin deficiency becomes complete in the majority of people with type 1 diabetes after 5 to 10 years of the disease. Exogenous insulin therapy is always needed and must be designed to mimic the normal pancreatic insulin release as closely as possible, with adjustments for meal size, timing, and composition as well as physical activity and conditioning. Careful scientific studies in nondiabetic adults have clearly shown a basal level of insulin secretion during periods of fasting and bursts of insulin release immediately with food ingestion. This immediate insulin release modulates the postprandial rise in plasma glucose so that it is minimal and returns to the premeal level within 2 hours, as insulin release ceases. Attendant with this action of insulin on glucose disposition are effects to suppress free fatty acid levels and to modulate amino acid disposition in a physiologic manner.

In type 1 diabetes, this normal physiology may be partially mimicked by a variety of approaches in which basal insulin is supplied and supplemented by premeal rapid-acting insulin. Presently, however, precise duplication of normal endogenous insulin secretion and action is not possible. The major reason is that insulin secreted by the pancreas enters the portal vein and acts on the liver in high concentrations to suppress hepatic glucose output. Hepatic degradation of insulin occurs and peripheral plasma insulin concentrations are substantially lower than portal levels. We are presently obliged to administer insulin subcutaneously in an unphysiologic manner, which leads to higher peripheral than portal insulin concentrations. Therefore, until more physiologic systems are developed for insulin administration, clinical attempts to return the altered metabolism of type 1 diabetes to normal will not be fully successful. Presently, no oral antidiabetic agent is effective in type 1 diabetes.

Insulin therapy must be tailored to each patient. For intensive glycemic

43

management, the type 1 diabetic patient and health care professionals must understand this conceptual framework and must be fully conversant with the actions of different insulin preparations and the effects of caloric intake, caloric expenditure, and other modifiers (including stress hormones, infection, and surgery) on glycemic response. For the type 1 diabetic patient, this understanding requires thorough education, which is repetitive and problem-solving in nature. Education is best accomplished by a team of well-versed health care professionals. The team approach is a prerequisite for successful intensive management in type 1 diabetes. Optimally, the team should consist of a physician diabetes specialist, a registered nurse who is a certified diabetes educator and specially trained as a team member for intensive management, and a nutritionist with similar background and training. A psychologist or counselor is included in comprehensive programs. Type 1 diabetes is a relatively rare disease, with less than 1 million patients in the United States.[7] Thus the concept of a team approach is feasible for most people in the U.S. with type 1 diabetes. It also is in accord with a major finding in the DCCT: the team approach is essential for successful management of people with type 1 diabetes.[14] In the section to follow and in the illustrative cases, a team approach is emphasized and utilized.

Medical Nutrition Therapy

Intensive management of type 1 diabetes requires initial and repetitive nutrition education and evaluation.[2,6] Although the overall goals of medical nutrition therapy are the same in people with type 1 and type 2 diabetes, the approaches are quite different. The goals are clear: (1) to achieve and maintain blood glucose and HbA1c values to as close to normal as is safely possible; (2) to achieve and maintain optimal plasma lipid or lipoprotein values; (3) to provide adequate calories for attaining and maintaining a reasonable weight and normal growth and development; and (4) to improve overall health through optimal nutrition.

Nutrition therapy must be individualized, according to food habits and lifestyle issues. An individualized nutritional plan begins with attention to usual dietary intake, including a dietary history with emphasis on serving sizes, methods of preparation, timing of meals, and consistency of patterns. This information is supplemented by a 24-hour recall form, which can be filled out at the first visit. Between visits, a food diary that records all ingested nutrients over a 2- to 3-day period is helpful.

The food plan must be integrated with insulin schedules and exercise patterns. Ideally, eating comparable meals from day to day at consistent times aids in insulin management of type 1 diabetes. Insulin types, dosages, and schedule must be integrated into the meal plan, with flexibility developed by experience and counseling. Self-monitoring of blood glucose before meals and at bedtime helps define patterns that may be addressed by dietary adjustments.

The literature about nutrition therapy for people with type 1 diabetes is extensive and may be contradictory and confusing. However, in recent years, particularly in the post-DCCT era of intensive glycemic management, there has been more general agreement on nutrition therapy for people with type 1 diabetes. Approximately 50–55% of calories should come from carbohydrate, 15–20% from protein, and 30% or less from fat. No more than 10% should come from saturated fat. Monounsaturated fat is used and replaces carbohydrate calories if hypertriglyceridemia is present. Fiber intake should be 20–35 gm/day from a variety of food sources. Caloric intake is adjusted to achieve and maintain optimal weight.

In many intensive management programs, carbohydrate counting is used. This system focuses on the grams of carbohydrate in each meal and allows the interchange of various carbohydrate exchanges for flexibility. Insulin coverage for the meal is adjusted according to carbohydrate counting. Special patient education about this system is required.

Intensive management of type 1 diabetes requires not only initial nutrition planning as described but also frequent evaluation and reinforcement. This goal is best accomplished by a registered dietician who is a certified diabetes educator and a regular member of the intensive management team.

Exercise

Regular exercise should be part of the therapeutic plan for people with type 1 diabetes who do not have advanced vascular complications.[1] It is important for the patient to recognize several key factors about exercise:

1. Acute exercise leads to an accelerated rate of fall of blood glucose if the pre-exercise level is normal (or slightly elevated) and insulin action is present.
2. Conversely, acute exercise is followed by a rise in plasma glucose and the possibility of ketosis if the pre-exercise blood glucose level is elevated and insulin action is waning.
3. Prolonged exercise not only may be associated with an acute fall in blood glucose in well-controlled patients, but its effect also may last 12–24 hours.

Tables 1 and 2 outline the recommendations for people with type 1 diabetes.

TABLE 1.   Management Strategies for Exercise in Type 1 Diabetes

- Monitor blood glucose before and after exercise.
- Learn the short- and longer-term responses to exercise.
- Delay exercise and take short-acting insulin if the blood glucose levels are > 250 mg/dl.
- Ingest added carbohydrate before exercise if glucose levels are < 100 mg/dl.
- Have carbohydrate-containing foods available during short-term and (especially) long-term exercise, and consume as needed if hypoglycemia occurs.
- Decrease the insulin dose that is expected to peak during exercise (i.e., prebreakfast intermediate insulin for exercise before supper). Reduction may be 10–30% or more, depending on duration and extent of exercise.
- Recognize that exercise may increase insulin release from either the arm or leg, if used as an injection site. Many health professionals recommend that only the abdomen be used for insulin injections.
- Table 2 gives some general guidelines for adjusting nutrient intake for exercise.

TABLE 2.   General Guidelines for Making Food Adjustments for Exercise

Type of Exercise and Examples	Blood Glucose (mg/dl)	Increase Food Intake by:	Suggestions of Food to Use
Exercise of short duration and low-to-moderate intensity	< 100	10–15 gm of carbohydrates per hour	1 fruit or 1 bread exchange
	100 or above	Not necessary to increase food	
Examples: Walking a half mile or leisurely bicycling for < 30 mins			
Exercise of moderate intensity	< 100	25–50 gm of carbohydrates before exercise, then 10–15 gm per hour of exercise	½ meat sandwich with a milk or fruit exchange
Examples: Tennis, swimming, jogging, bicycling, gardening, golfing or vacuuming	100–175	10–15 gm of carbohydrates per hour of exercise	1 fruit or 1 bread exchange
	175–225	Not necessary to increase food	
	≥ 225	Do not begin exercise until blood glucose is under better control	
Strenuous exercise	< 100	50 gm of carbohydrates; monitor blood glucose carefully	1 meat sandwich (2 slices of bread) with a milk and fruit exchange

TABLE 2. General Guidelines for Making Food Adjustments for Exercise (Continued)			
Type of Exercise and Examples	Blood Glucose (mg/dl)	Increase Food Intake by:	Suggestions of Food to Use
Examples: Football, hockey, racquetball or basketball games; strenuous bicycling shoveling heavy snow	100–175	25–50 mg of carbohydrates, depending on intensity and duration	½ meat sandwich with a milk or fruit exchange
	175–225	10–15 gm of carbohydrates per hour of exercise	1 fruit or 1 bread exchange
	≥ 225	Not necessary to increase food Insulin may be needed	

In summary, the person with type 1 diabetes must recognize the importance of exercise as part of the therapeutic plan and be prepared to regularly act after checking these key issues before exercise:

- Duration and intensity of planned exercise.
- Insulin schedule: timing, site of injection dose.
- Food intake, prior to and during exercise.
- Blood glucose, prior to and after exercise.
- Urine ketones, if BG > 250mg/dl.

Insulin Preparations

A wide variety of insulin preparations is available for therapy with insulin in type 1 diabetic patients. The preparations are either human insulin produced by recombinant DNA technology or insulin analogs, in which the insulin molecule is altered to provide an immediate onset of action or a long-acting, virtually peakless action. A comparison of the onset, peak, and duration of action of rapid, short, intermediate, and long-acting human insulins and analogs is shown in Table 3.

Careful scrutiny of Table 3 indicates that a variety of insulin combinations theoretically can be used in people with type 1 diabetes to replace the absent endogenous insulin supply. Conceptually, however, insulin should be prescribed in a fashion that most closely mimics the secretion of insulin in the fasting and fed state by the pancreas of a person who does not have diabetes. There should be a relatively constant basal 24-hour insulin supply that is supplemented by rapid- or short-acting insulin taken before or at mealtime as a bolus injection.

TABLE 3.	Comparison Actions of Human Insulins and Analogs		
Insulin Preparation	Onset of Action	Peak Action	Duration of Action
Lispro*/Aspart*	5–15 minutes	1–2 hours	4–6 hours
Human regular	30–60 minutes	2–4 hours	6–10 hours
Human NPH/lente	1–2 hours	4–8 hours	10–18 hours
Ultralente	2–4 hours	8–14 hours	18–24 hours
Glargine*	1–2 hours	Flat	24 hours
*Insulin analog.			

Basal Insulin Supply

Basal insulin supply can best be achieved either by infusion of rapid-acting insulin at a constant rate by an insulin pump or by using a bed-time injection of insulin glargine. Generally, about 50–60% of total insulin requirements should be basal insulin, and approximately 40–50% should be premeal insulin. In the DCCT, patients randomized into the intensive management group required 0.73 u/kg as an average total dose. A typical safe starting basal rate is 0.3 u/kg/24 hr. Basal rate is adjusted to produce FBG levels of 80–120 mg/dl.

In the past, when long-acting, peakless insulin preparations were not available, physicians tried to supply basal insulin in a variety of ways. A popular technique was to give ultralente insulin in equal doses before breakfast and supper and use rapid- or short-acting insulin before meals. The rapid/short-acting insulin was mixed with ultralente just before injection. This technique is effective in some patients but may result in peaking of the ultralente and hypoglycemia at times of peak action (8–14 hours). A second strategy to provide basal insulin coverage is the use of an intermediate insulin at bedtime, targeting the first prebreakfast blood glucose to evaluate the dosage. This technique also may lead to early-morning hypoglycemia in view of the time course of action of the intermediate insulin. Late injection (i.e., 11 p.m. or later) with a bedtime protein snack often avoids this problem. Finally, one can try to provide basal insulin by two doses of intermediate insulin (before breakfast and at bedtime). However, in type 1 diabetic patients this strategy is often complicated by presupper and/or early-morning hypoglycemia as one strives for intensive management goals.

Studies have demonstrated that people with type 1 diabetes have close to optimal glycemic control with the fewest episodes of hypoglycemia when basal insulin supply is provided either by rapid-acting insulin by an infusion pump or by insulin glargine injected at bedtime.[9] For individual patients, however, trials of other regimens using ultralente or intermediate-acting insulins may be successful.

Bolus Insulin Doses

There is an immediate release of insulin from the normally functioning pancreas as it senses an ingested nutrient supply. This insulin-secretion curve is most closely matched by subcutaneous injection of either the lispro or aspart insulin analogue. Studies have shown that with careful dosage titration, postprandial glucose levels are lower with these analogs than with a comparable dose of short-acting regular insulin. In an attempt to mimic the physiologic insulin rise, regular insulin should be given 30 minutes before the meal, whereas the rapid-acting insulins are given at the time of eating.

Because the rapid-acting insulins have a duration of action that is shorter than regular insulin, there may be a rise in blood glucose before the next meal—particularly if it is eaten 4 hours or more after the previous meal. In this case, there are several options. First, one can raise the rapid-acting insulin dose or give it during the meal. Preliminary studies have suggested that aspart insulin may have a slightly longer duration of action than lispro insulin, and this switch may be effective. Regular insulin may be substituted for the rapid-acting insulin to give a longer duration of action, with the potential problem of less rapid onset of action. Finally, if escape from the rapid-acting insulin action continues to occur before the following meal, one should increase the basal insulin dosage (or rate of infusion by pump) to achieve improved premeal glycemic control.

Glucose Monitoring

With these intensive management schemes, it is critical that the type 1 diabetic patient be adept and accurate with self-monitoring of blood glucose. Various excellent glucose monitors have been developed, and every type 1 diabetic patient should regularly monitor blood glucose levels to gauge insulin, diet, and exercise regimens. Because the rapid- or short-acting insulin is given before each of the three main meals, most physicians advise patients to check blood glucose at these times. Insulin doses are adjusted depending on the blood glucose level, portion size, and carbohydrate content of the meal and the patient's exercise schedule. Periodic monitoring of 1–2 hour postprandial blood glucose levels after different meals is very useful. Typical scenarios in type 1 diabetics are given in the case presentations.

As previously stressed, intensive management of this type is best handled by a diabetes team, consisting of a physician specializing in intensive diabetic management, a nurse who is also a certified diabetes educator (CDE) and experienced in this discipline, and a similarly trained dietician. A team member must be available at all times to interrelate with patients, who may communicate management issues by telephone, facsimile, e-mail, or letter. Team management must be coordinated with general medical care provided by the primary care physician.

Key Points: Intensive Glucose Management of Type 1 Diabetes

- ⊙ A major concept in providing insulin therapy for people with type 1 diabetes is to provide 50–60% of the total dose as basal insulin and the remainder as premeal rapid- or short-acting insulin.
- ⊙ Average total insulin requirement for intensive management in type 1 diabetes is approximately 0.7 U/kg/24 hours.
- ⊙ Insulin therapy must be tailored for each type 1 diabetic, with close coordination with meal plan and exercise program.
- ⊙ Repetitive visits with a dietician are needed to develop successful medical nutrition therapy.
- ⊙ Acute exercise in type 1 diabetes may be followed by hyperglycemia (if insulin action is decreasing) or hypoglycemia (if insulin action is increasing). Hypoglycemia may be delayed 12–24 hours, especially after strenuous exercise and conditioning in well-controlled patients.
- ⊙ Blood glucose should be measured before and after exercise and different approaches used (caloric adjustment vs. change in insulin dose) until the right combination for that patient is achieved.
- ⊙ A wide variety of insulin preparations is available. Basal insulin is most accurately supplied by a bedtime injection of insulin glargine or by insulin infusion pump. Alternatively, ultralente may be given in equal doses before breakfast and supper or intermediate insulin at bedtime (late, with a protein snack).
- ⊙ Meals are best covered by a simultaneous injection of a rapid-acting insulin analog: insulin lispro or aspart. If action is too short to cover blood glucose before the next meal, regular insulin (30 min a.c.) or raising the basal insulin dosage may be sucessful.
- ⊙ If the HbA1c does not agree with the blood glucose log, believe the HbA1c.
- ⊙ If no progress is made after trying a schedule for 2–3 months, it is wise to start all over again with a different intensive management scheme. This strategy gets everybody's attention.
- ⊙ Memory meters are useful devices to check accuracy of the written records of patients.
- ⊙ The abdomen should be used for insulin injections. Rates of absorption vary too much from arms and legs, especially for people who exercise.

Key Points: (*Continued*)

- Insulin pens are useful for many type 1 diabetics.
- The dietician should be an integral part of the team. Changes in diet, exercise, and insulin must be coordinated and evaluated.
- A counselor can do wonders for problem patients and frazzled medical staff.
- When spikes of high preprandial glucose levels are mingled with many low-to-normal levels, these spikes usually are of dietary origin.
- If the fasting blood glucose level is brought to normal, management for the rest of the day is improved.
- Use glucose (tablets of 4–5 grams each) for mild hypoglycemia. Measure blood glucose after 1, 2, or 3 of the tablets until it is in normal range. The goal is to titrate glucose levels to the normal range.
- If hypoglycemia is the problem, missed or delayed meals and/or exercise may be the problem. If the patient is on a regimen with 70% or more of the total insulin as intermediate insulin, this is more likely the culprit rather than the short-acting insulin.
- If 3 a.m. hypoglycemia is the problem with presupper intermediate insulin, it should be shifted to 11 p.m. or later. Raise the amount of protein in the bedtime snack.
- Significant others should be aware of the patient's intensive management plan.
- A pharmacist trained in diabetes management can help with intensive insulin therapy and monitoring.
- Intensive management should be done by a health care team that includes a physician, diabetes nurse clinician (CDE), a dietician (CDE), and optimally a clinical counselor.

Future Strategies and Special Issues

Inhaled Insulin

Insulin in a powdered form has been shown in clinical trials to be effective if it is inhaled under controlled conditions.[8,13] In one system, delivery is by aerosol, and insulin is contained in a blister within the aerosol device. An air-assist mechanism dispenses the powdered insulin into a cloud that is captured in a holding chamber and then inhaled by the patient. The doses can be adjusted to deliver 3–18 units (in 3-unit increments) into the systemic circulation after absorption from the alveoli. Preliminary studies in type 1 and in type 2 diabetic patients have shown efficacy comparable to that of rapid-acting insulin.[4,13] Large quantities of powdered insulin (approximately 10 times the subcutaneous dose) must be used when insulin is administered by aerosol. Patient satisfaction is generally high; however, the early devices are quite bulky to use and to carry around. Long-term controlled trials of safety (especially pulmonary) and efficacy in type 1 and type 2 diabetes are under way. This is a promising method for diabetic patients to take premeal insulin without the need for subcutaneous injections. If long-term efficacy and safety are shown and user-friendly devices are developed, inhaled powder will be a major advance in insulin therapy.

Pancreas Transplantation

Currently, the guideline for pancreas transplantation in patients with type 1 diabetes limits the procedure to diabetic patients with end-stage renal disease who have had or are scheduled to have a kidney transplant.[3] Including a pancreas transplant with a renal transplant often restores normal glycemia and may help to prolong kidney survival. Evidence indicates that pancreas transplantation can reverse the lesions of diabetic nephropathy if it results in 5 years or more of normoglycemia.[5] Pancreas transplantation that is done simultaneously with kidney transplantation is preferable, but transplantation also may be done after a kidney transplant.

In a few specialized centers, whole-organ pancreas transplantation is performed in the absence of indications for a kidney transplant. ADA guidelines include (1) a history of frequent, severe, acute metabolic complications requiring medical attention; (2) severe, incapacitating clinical and emotional problems with exogenous insulin therapy; and (3) consistent failure of insulin management to prevent acute complications.

Pancreatic islet cell transplantation, with injection directly into the liver, is a research procedure. Recent developments in harvesting adequate numbers of pancreatic islets from cadaver pancreases and revised immunologic suppression techniques that use no corticosteroids have yielded exciting short-term results.[10,12] Large-scale research trials are under way at many centers, and this transplantation technique holds great promise for future success for selected type 1 diabetic patients.

Amylin

Amylin, a peptide first identified in the pancreatic islets by Opie in 1901, is a 37-amino acid neuroendocrine peptide genetically related to calcitonin. It has been called islet amyloid polypeptide (IAPP). The precursor of IAPP is transferred in the pancreatic islets, along with proinsulin to the Golgi apparatus. The precursor is processed by the same enzymatic machinery as proinsulin to release IAPP. It is then stored in the insulin granules and released along with insulin. IAPP secretion is stimulated by glucose; IAPP amounts to less than 5% of the amount of insulin released in vitro at high glucose concentrations.

IAPP slows gastric emptying and may cause vasodilation. The effects of amylin are mediated through the central nervous system. There are specific amylin-binding sites in the area postrema of the brain. Outflow is via efferent pathways of the vagus nerve.[11] People with type 1 diabetes have an absolute deficiency of amylin. In view of this deficiency and the pharmacologic properties of amylin, amylin replacement may be an effective clinical management tool to supplement the action of insulin in type 1 diabetes.

Pramlintide acetate is a synthetic analog with activities like those of amylin. In type 1 diabetes, subcutaneous injections before meals decreases postprandial glucagon secretion, delays gastric emptying, and slows the delivery of oral nutrients into the small intestine. Gastric emptying may be delayed 1–1½ hours. The result is a decrease in postprandial hyperglycemia. Although glucagon secretion is decreased, the pancreatic glucagon response to hypoglycemia is normal, as is the response of other glucose counterregulatory hormones.

A number of phase III studies have been reported in type 1 diabetes and reviewed by the Food and Drug Administration (FDA). Amylin (Symlin TM or pramLintide acetate) is proposed as adjunctive therapy to insulin for the treatment of people with type 1 diabetes. Suppression of glucagon secretion, slowing of the rate of nutrient delivery, and suppression of appetite are viewed as positive adjuncts to insulin action.

In phase III studies in type 2 diabetes, modest reductions in HbA1c (up to 0.4% vs. placebo) are seen when pramlintide is given with insulin therapy.[15] Weight loss usually occurs, and appetite often is decreased. Major side effects are nausea and an increased incidence of hypoglycemia. Initial studies required up to four premeal subcutaneous injections; plans are to overcome this problem with long-acting preparations, which are presently in phase II development.

References

1. American Diabetes Association: Diabetes mellitus and exercise. Diabetes Care 25:S64–S68, 2002.
2. American Diabetes Association: Evidence-based nutrition principles and recommendations for the treatment and prevention of diabetes and related complications. Diabetes Care 25:S50–S60, 2002.
3. American Diabetes Association: Pancreas transplantation for patients with type 1 diabetes. Diabetes Care 25:S111, 2002.
4. Cefalu WT, Skyler JS, Kourides IA, et al: Inhaled human insulin treatment in patients with type II diabetes mellitus. Ann Intern Med 134:203–207, 2001.
5. Fioretto P, Steffes MW, Sutherland DER, et al: Reversal of lesions of diabetic nephropathy after pancreas transplantation. N Engl J Med 339:69–75, 1998.
6. Franz MJ, Bantle JP, Beebe CA, et al: Evidence-based nutrition principles and recommendations for the treatment and prevention of diabetes and related complications. Diabetes Care 25:148–198, 2002.

7. LaPorte RE, Matsushima M, Chang YF: Prevalence and incidence of insulin-dependent diabetes. In Diabetes in America, 2nd Edition. National Institutes of Health, National Institute of Diabetes and Digestive and Kidney Disease. NIH Publication No. 95–1468. 1995, pp 37–45.

8. Nathan D, et al: Inhaled insulin for type 2 diabetes: Solution or Distraction? [editorial]. Ann Intern Med 134:242–244, 2001.

9. Ratner RE, Hirsch IB, Neifing JL, et al: Less hypoglycemia with insulin glargine in intensive insulin therapy for type 1 diabetes. U.S. Study Group of Insulin Glargine in Type 1 Diabetes. Diabetes Care 23:639–643, 2000.

10. Robertson RP: Successful islet transplantation for patients with diabetes—fact or fantasy? N Engl J Med 343:289–290, 2000.

11. Samson M, Szarka LA, Camilleri M, et al: Pramlintide, an amylin analog, selectively delays gastric emptying: Potential role of vagal inhibition. Am J Physiol Gastrointest Liver Physiol 278:G946–951, 2000.

12. Shapiro AMJ, Lakey JRT, Ryan EA, et al: Islet transplantation in seven patients with type 1 diabetes mellitus using a glucocorticoid-free immunosuppressive regimen. N Engl J Med 343:230–238, 2000.

13. Skyler JS, Cefalu WT, Kourides IA, et al: Efficacy of inhaled human insulin in type 1 diabetes mellitus: A randomised proof-of-concept study. Lancet 357:331–335, 2001.

14. The Diabetes Control and Complications Trial Research Group: The effect of intensive treatment of diabetes on the development and progression of long-term complications in insulin-dependent diabetes mellitus. N Engl J Med 329:977–986, 1993.

15. Thompson RG, Pearson L, Schoenfeld SL, et al: Pramlintide, a synthetic analog of human amylin, improves the metabolic profile of patients with type 2 diabetes using insulin. The Pramlintide in Type 2 Diabetes Group. Diabetes Care 21:987–993, 1998.

Intensive Management of Special Issues in Type 1 Diabetes

chapter
6

Nephropathy

Natural History

At the time of diagnosis of type 1 diabetes, renal blood flow (RBF) and glomerular filtration rate (GFR) are often elevated, but histologic changes on renal biopsy are not present. Within 3 years, however, findings include an increase in the mesangial matrix and thickening of the capillary basement membrane of the renal glomeruli.[24] Over the next 10–20 years histologic changes progress, and microalbuminuria (30–300 mg albumin/24 hr) occurs in 30–40% of type 1 diabetic patients treated with conventional therapy. Intensive glycemic management reduces this risk by about 40–50%.[31,37] If the patient continues with standard medical therapy, microalbuminuria increases to clinical proteinuria (> 300 mg albumin/24 hr) and the elevated RBF and GFR fall to normal or below normal. Without modern therapy, about 50% of patients progress to end-stage renal disease (ESRD) with a 50% decrease in GFR in about 5 years, then to ESRD requiring dialysis and/or transplantation within the next 3 years. An elevation of blood pressure > 130/80 mmHg usually occurs at the time of microalbuminuria, and clinical hypertension (BP ≥ 140/90 mmHg) is seen in most patients at the stage of clinical proteinuria.[12,13,20,25]

Concomitant with this process is often a shift in the lipoprotein profile, with a rise in LDL cholesterol and triglycerides and a fall in HDL cholesterol. This combination of an atherogenic lipoprotein profile and hypertension is a major contributor to accelerated atherosclerosis in type 1 diabetics with nephropathy. Prospective, long-term studies of type 1 diabetic patients in Finland have shown that nephropathy has a major impact on the atherosclerotic complications of coronary heart disease and stroke.[40] Virtually no cases of cardiovascular disease were clinically apparent before 12 years of duration of type 1 diabetes (Fig. 1). However, the cumulative incidence of cardiovascular disease by age 40 was 43% in type 1 patients with nephropathy, but only 7% in those without

Figure 1. Cumulative incidence of coronary heart disease (CHD), stroke, and all cardiovascular disease (CVD) in type 1 diabetic subjects (n = 4702) with (*dotted line*) and without diabetic nephropathy (*solid line,* n = 446) by duration of diabetes. (From Tuomilehto J, et al: Diabetologia 41:784–790, 1998, with permission. Copyright© Springer-Verlag, 1998.)

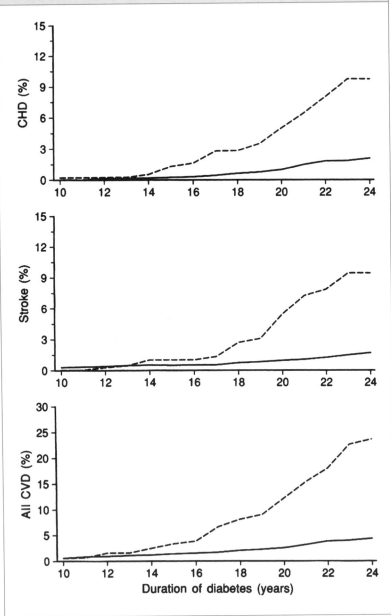

nephropathy. The risk of coronary heart disease or stroke was increased 10-fold by the presence of nephropathy.

Nephropathy and the associated increased cardiovascular risk has traditionally been the major contributor to mortality in type 1 diabetes. Fortunately, modern therapy with close attention to control of glucose, hypertension, microalbuminuria, and lipoprotein alterations has greatly modified this natural history. In 1971, it was reported that 75–80% of type 1 diabetic patients with a 10-year duration of nephropathy were dead.[14] By 1985, this figure was approximately 40%.[15] In a 1996 study, cumulative mortality was down to 20% in 10 years.[25] However, the cumulative incidence of CHD, stroke, and all CVD with increasing duration of type 1 diabetes continues to be greater in patients with nephropathy than in those without nephropathy (Fig. 1). These figures probably will continue to improve in the next few decades because of exciting findings from a variety of collaborative controlled trials of glycemic regulation, hypertension control, inhibitors of angiotensin II synthesis and/or action, and treatment of microalbuminuria.

Preserving Renal Function

Glucose Control. As previously discussed, intensive glycemic management in the DCCT reduced the occurrence of microalbuminuria ($\geq$ 40 mg/24 hr) by 39% and the occurrences of albuminuria ($\geq$ 300 mg/24 hr) by 54%.[37] Analysts of 3- to 4-year follow-up data revealed that microalbuminuria occurred in 11% of the former conventional therapy group but in only 5% in the former intensive therapy group (53% odds reduction).[31]

In Sweden, a declining incidence of nephropathy has been seen with long-term follow-up of people with type 1 diabetes.[7] A decrease was seen in the incidence of persistent clinical albuminuria (300 mg by dipstick) after 15–20 years of type 1 diabetes from 28% (1961–1965 cohort) to 0% (1976–1980 cohort). The incidence of microalbuminuria, which is not detected by dipstick, was not reported. The findings were concomitant with a HbA1c level of 7.1% in patients without albuminuria vs. 8.1% in those with albuminuria. Reversal of diabetic renal histopathology after 10 years of normoglycemia after pancreas transplantation has been reported.

Thus, intensive glycemic management is a critical component of the approach to preserving renal function in people with type 1 diabetes. Nevertheless, microalbuminuria may occur in spite of intensive glycemic management, and adjunctive therapy is indicated.

Microalbuminuria. Glomerular hyperfiltration and intraglomerular hypertension are associated with microalbuminuria, and their reduction decreases urinary albumin excretion. In the 1980s, studies in animals by

Brenner's group showed that angiotensin-converting enzyme (ACE) inhibitors normalized intraglomerular hypertension by reducing efferent arteriolar pressure. The progression of diabetic nephropathy was retarded.[8]

In people with type 1 diabetes, microalbuminuria has been shown to be a predictor of nephropathy progression.[20,21,22,25,26,27,43] Controlled clinical trials have demonstrated that therapy with ACE inhibitors leads to regression of the microalbuminuria and markedly delays the progression to clinical albuminuria and/or end-stage renal failure.[10,16,19,23,30,38,44] Long-term beneficial effects are seen. Eight years of ACE inhibitor therapy in type 1 patients with microalbuminuria has been shown to preserve normal renal function.

An elevation of blood pressure often occurs with development of microalbuminuria, and untreated hypertension clearly accelerates progression of nephropathy.[20,25] ACE inhibitor therapy for hypertension is a standard of care in diabetes. Furthermore, it is now established that ACE inhibitor therapy for microalbuminuria lowers urinary albumin excretion and slows progression of nephropathy in normotensive patients.[28] The current standard of care is to start ACE inhibitor therapy when microalbuminuria and/or BP > 130/80 mmHg is first recognized in people with type 1 diabetes rather than waiting until a BP ≥ 140/90 mmHg develops.

Studies are under way to determine whether ACE inhibitor therapy prevents microalbuminuria in patients destined to develop it. Because microalbuminuria occurs in only 30–40% of people with type 1 diabetes and because we presently have no genetic (or other) markers, it is not indicated to start all type 1 patients on ACE inhibitor therapy. Future studies will help define patients at risk and may show a beneficial effect of ACE inhibitor therapy before microalbuminuria occurs.

In short-term studies of 3 years' duration, no effect of ACE inhibitor on diabetic histopathologic renal damage has been seen in normotensive type 1 diabetic patients with micro- or macroalbuminuria.[18,29,39] It appears that a new study with large sample size, a narrow albuminuria and GFR range, less advanced glomerular structural changes and a longer duration of effective doses of ACE inhibitor therapy is indicated to determine clearly whether renal structure can be altered by ACE inhibitor therapy.

It is generally accepted that the angiotensin receptor blockers (ARBs) will prove to be equally effective as ACE inhibitor therapy. Large-scale controlled studies in type 1 diabetic patients, however, are limited. Presently ARB therapy is recommended for type 1 diabetic patients with microalbuminuria who are allergic to ACE inhibitor therapy or who develop an uncontrollable cough while being treated with ACE inhibitors. Use of ARBs in type 2 diabetes is discussed in another chapter.

Albuminuria. Clinically significant albuminuria is defined as the excretion of ≥300 mg albumin/24 hours. In type 1 diabetes, it is a sign of late-stage nephropathy, as previously noted, and usually is accompanied by a falling GFR, hypertension, and an atherogenic lipid profile and cardiovascular disease. Early studies of ACE inhibitor therapy in type 1 diabetic patients with nephropathy were done in this group. In the classic trial by Lewis et al., captopril treatment was associated with a 48% reduction in the risk of a doubling of serum creatinine and a 50% reduction in the risk of the combined endpoints of death, dialysis, and transplantation compared with placebo therapy (Fig. 2).[16] The effects were independent of a small disparity in blood pressure between the two groups, suggesting that the mechanism was not dependent on the antihypertensive action of captopril. Urinary albumin excretion was reduced in the captopril-treated group. ACE inhibitors may reduce progression of cardiovascular disease by effects on endothelial function or other mechanisms.[11]

Key Points: Nephropathy

- ☞ Nephropathy has traditionally occurred in 30–40% of people with type 1 diabetes.
- ☞ Mortality from complications of nephropathy in type 1 diabetes was 80% in 1971, 40% in 1984, and 20% in 1996.
- ☞ With modern intensive management of glucose, blood pressure, albuminuria, and the synthesis and/or action of angiotensin II, the incidence of nephropathy and its cardiovascular complications will continue to decrease.
- ☞ Intensive glucose management, with a HbA1c goal of < 7%, will decrease occurrence of microalbuminuria and subsequent diabetic nephropathy.
- ☞ If microalbuminuria (> 30 mg/24 hr) is present, therapy with angiotensin-converting enzyme inhibitors leads to regression of microalbuminuria and delays the progression to clinical albuminuria (≥ 300 mg/24 hr) and/or end-stage renal failure.
- ☞ These effects are seen in normotensive as well as hypertensive type 1 diabetic patients with microalbuminuria.
- ☞ ACE inhibitor therapy in type 1 diabetic patients with clinical albuminuria and an elevated serum creatinine leads to a 48–50% reduction in the risk of doubling of serum creatinine or progression to end-stage renal disease

Hypertension

In the discussion of preserving renal function in people with type 1 diabetes, we have concentrated on intensive glycemic regulation and

Figure 2. Cumulative incidence of events in patients with diabetic nephropathy in the captopril and placebo groups. Panel A shows the cumulative percentage of patients with the primary end point: a doubling of the base-line serum creatinine concentration to at least 2.0 mg/dl. Panel B shows the cumulative percentage of patients who died or required dialysis or renal transplantation. The numbers at the bottom of each panel are the numbers of patients in each group at risk for the event at base line and after each 6-month period. (From Lewis E, et al: N Eng J Med 329:1456–1462, 1993, with permission. Copyright©1993, Massachusetts Medical Society. All rights reserved.)

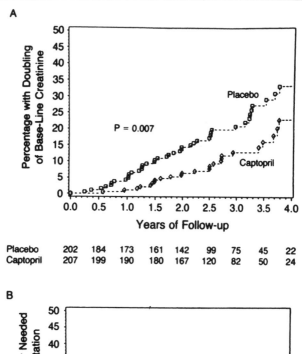

Placebo	202	184	173	161	142	99	75	45	22
Captopril	207	199	190	180	167	120	82	50	24

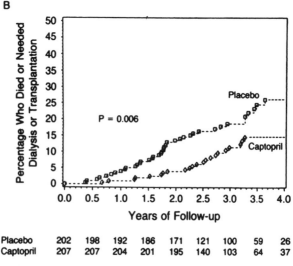

Placebo	202	198	192	186	171	121	100	59	26
Captopril	207	207	204	201	195	140	103	64	37

treatment of the renin-angiotensin system. The other major variable to consider is the management of hypertension in type 1 diabetes.

The majority of patients with type 1 diabetes are normotensive until microalbuminuria develops.[20,25] Of course, hypertension unrelated to nephropathy can occur but does not exceed the prevalence in the general population. At the stage of microalbuminuria, the blood pressure in type 1 diabetes usually exceeds 130/80 mmHg but may stay below the older standard of < 140/90 mmHg. At the stage of established diabetic nephropathy (urinary albumin ≥ 300 mg/day), the majority of people with type 1 diabetes have hypertension, and virtually all have hypertension at the point of end-stage renal disease.

Therapy for hypertension slows the progression of retinal and renal disease and prevents cardiovascular events in type 1 diabetes. Presently, a consensus has been reached that antihypertensive therapy should have a goal of < 130/80 mmHg.[3,4,5,6] Thus, many physicians start ACE inhibitor (or ARB) therapy at blood pressure levels of 130/80 mmHg in type 1 diabetes. As the disease progresses, escape from this ideal goal frequently occurs, and a second agent is added. With further progression of nephropathy, particularly at the stage of renal failure or ESRD, combinations of three or more agents may be required (i.e., thiazides, calcium channel blockers, beta blockers).

Much information about the effect of therapy for hypertension comes from large-scale trials in type 2 rather than type 1 diabetes. For this reason, a thorough discussion of the evidence in support of aggressive antihypertensive therapy, as well as recommended techniques to achieve goals, is included in the section on type 2 diabetes. In type 1 diabetes, a focus on treatment of hypertension as it occurs with the development of microalbuminuria and/or nephropathy is the most critical issue. The evidence in support of aggressive therapy is very strong.

Key Points: Hypertension

- ⇨ At the stage of microalbuminuria, there is usually a rise in blood pressure in type 1 diabetes.
- ⇨ Antihypertensive therapy, with ACE inhibitor or ARB should be started when BP is ≥130/80 mmHg in type 1 diabetes.
- ⇨ Virtually all type 1 patients with clinical albuminuria have BP ≥130/80 mmHg.
- ⇨ Therapy for hypertension slows the progression of renal disease and prevents cardiovascular events in type 1 diabetes.
- ⇨ The goal of therapy is BP ≤ 130/80 mmHg.

Key Points: (*Continued*)

↪ As nephropathy progresses, there is usually a need for the addition of a second or third (or more) antihypertensive agent to provide adequate blood pressure control.

↪ The following agents are effective in treating blood pressure elevation in type 1 diabetes: ACE inhibitors, ARBs, thiazides, calcium channel blockers, and cardiospecific beta blockers. In selected patients, combinations, including other agents, may be necessary.

Lipids/Lipoproteins

In well-controlled type 1 diabetes not complicated by nephropathy, plasma lipid or lipoprotein levels are usually normal. For instance, on entry into the DCCT, participants had lipid profiles that were the same as similarly aged nondiabetics.[33] As already noted, nephropathy is usually associated with the development of an atherogenic lipid profile, which contributes to a 25-fold increase in cardiovascular disease in the setting of established diabetic nephropathy.

Glycemic regulation is another important factor that determines the plasma lipid/lipoprotein profile in type 1 diabetes. Before the DCCT, short-term studies in type 1 diabetics with markedly elevated HbA1c levels (>12%) showed that poor glycemic control was associated with elevations in plasma cholesterol, LDL-cholesterol, triglycerides, and low plasma HDL-cholesterol concentrations. These values were reversed toward normal by short-term glycemic regulation on an inpatient basis.[17] Cross-sectional studies showed a similar trend. In the DCCT, cholesterol, LDL cholesterol, and triglyceride levels were significantly lower in the intensively treated than in the conventionally treated group.[33] Intensive therapy lowered the risk of developing LDL-C levels >160 mg/dl by 54% and >130 mg/dl by 27% in the secondary prevention group. This group entered the trial with moderate nonproliferative retinopathy and a duration of type 1 diabetes of 1–15 years. A minority of patients had microalbuminuria when they entered the trial.

Of interest, however, the mean LDL-C levels in the intensively treated and the conventionally treated patients in both cohorts in the DCCT were above the level of 100 mg/dl and below 130 mg/dl. Furthermore, although it was not a significant difference, there was a trend toward a decrease in the number of macrovascular events in the intensively treated group (23 events) vs. the conventionally treated group (40 events). Current guidelines for care indicate an LDL-C goal of 100 mg/dl or below; however, these guidelines are based on large-scale randomized trials in type 2 diabetes or in nondiabetic subjects. Goals for triglycerides and HDL-C suffer from a similar lack of prospective trial data in type 1 diabetes. However, these variables are quite responsive to intensive glycemic regulation in most type 1 diabetics thus the current guidelines, as previously described, appear to be adequate.

Key Points: Lipids/Lipoproteins

- ◌ When type 1 diabetes is not under poor glycemic control (i.e., HbA1c > 12%), plasma lipid and lipoprotein levels are usually within normal limits.
- ◌ Intensive glycemic control leads to a slight fall in cholesterol, LDL cholesterol, and triglycerides and a rise in HDL cholesterol.
- ◌ In the DCCT, with intensive glycemic management, mean LDL-C levels were between 100 and 130 mg/dl.
- ◌ An LDL-C goal of < 100 mg/dl is accepted as the guideline for people with diabetes; however, data are primarily from trials in type 2 diabetes.
- ◌ With the development of albuminuria, a shift to an atherogenic lipid profile is usually seen: elevated LDL-C, cholesterol, and triglycerides and a low HDL-C.
- ◌ The combination of this lipid profile with hypertension is a major contributor to the increased cardiovascular risk in type 1 diabetes.
- ◌ Aggressive treatment with lipid therapeutic agents (e.g., statins, fibrates) often is needed to achieve low-risk lipid/lipoprotein goals in type 1 patients with nephropathy.

Retinopathy

Most people with type 1 diabetes have retinopathy as the duration of the disease increases.[1] Visual impairment and blindness may occur. Intensive glycemic regulation prevents or slows the development of clinically significant changes in patients without retinopathy and delays progression in patients with nonproliferative retinopathy.[31,36,37] Early worsening of retinopathy after rapid control of blood glucose may occur, particularly in type 1 diabetic patients with advanced retinopathy and diabetes of long duration. This phenomenon was studied in the DCCT,[32,36] where it was noted in some patients in the intensive therapy group with longstanding poor glycemic control and retinopathy at or past the moderate nonproliferative stage. Early worsening (at 6 or 12 months) occurred in 13.1% of the intensive treatment group vs. 7.6% of the conventional therapy group (p < 0.001). Recovery occurred by 18 months in the majority of these patients, but five progressed to high-risk proliferative retinopathy or clinically significant macular edema. All responded to laser therapy.

Thus, in patients whose retinopathy is approaching the high-risk stage, ophthalmologic evaluation should be sought, and the initiation of intensive glycemic management should be delayed until photocoagulation is completed. This strategy is particularly prudent in type 1 patients with a history of a long duration of poor glycemic control.

It is well established that hypertension is a risk factor for diabetic maculopathy and proliferative diabetic retinopathy. The relative risk of maculopathy is increased eightfold and the risk of proliferative retinopathy fivefold with increasing diastolic pressure. Beneficial effects of antihypertensive therapy on the progression of nephropathy are clear. It is likely that intensive blood pressure-lowering also decreases the risk of advancing retinopathy in type 1 diabetes. The best data from a large-scale collaborative trial, however, come from the UKPDS, a study in type 2 diabetes. A policy of tight blood pressure control was associated with a 37% reduction in retinopathy.[41,42] Thus, intensive blood pressure- and blood glucose-lowering are important strategies to prevent or delay progression of diabetic retinopathy.

ACE inhibitors appear to slow progression of diabetic retinopathy. This benefit is not necessarily caused by blood pressure-lowering or glycemic regulation. In the EURODIAB controlled trial of lisinopril in insulin-dependent diabetes mellitus (EUCLID) study,[9,38] nonproliferative retinopathy progressed by at least 1 level in 2 years in 13.2% of patients on lisinopril, but in 23.4% in the control group of type 1 diabetic patients (50% reduction, p = 0.02). The majority of these patients did not have microalbuminuria, and the protective effect was not dependent on the presence of microalbumin in the urine. Patients with better glycemic control had the most benefit from ACE inhibitor therapy, suggesting that this combination is the best approach. The effects of ACE inhibitor therapy on retinopathy did not appear to be due to blood pressure reduction, and a direct effect on retinal blood flow was suggested. These results are similar to those reported in other, smaller studies in type 1 and type 2 diabetes. Thus, ACE inhibitor therapy may decrease retinopathy progression in nonhypertensive type 1 diabetic patients with little or no nephropathy. Confirmatory trials, however, are needed before these results are translated to clinical practice guidelines.

Key Points: Retinopathy

- ∞ The incidence of retinopathy approaches 100% in people with type 1 diabetes after 15–20 years of standard management.
- ∞ Intensive glycemic management, with a HbA1c goal of ≤ 7%, may decrease the rate of progression to clinically significant retinopathy in type 1 subjects without retinopathy.

Key Points: (*Continued*)

↪ In type 1 patients with preproliferative retinopathy, rate of progression to clinically significant retinopathy is markedly decreased by intensive glycemic management.

↪ For every 1% decrease of HbA1c, the risk of progression of retinopathy is decreased about 25% in type 1 diabetes.

↪ Early worsening of diabetic retinopathy may be seen with intensive glycemic management, particularly in type 1 diabetic patients with moderate nonproliferative retinopathy and a long history of poor glycemic control.

↪ Ophthalmologic evaluation is indicated in such patients before intensive glycemic control is instituted to evaluate the need for photocoagulation therapy.

↪ Hypertension is an added risk factor for progression of diabetic retinopathy, maculopathy and/or proliferative retinopathy. Beneficial effects of antihypertensive therapy are clear.

↪ ACE inhibitor therapy appears to have a special protective effect on retinopathy progression in addition to effects on blood pressure control.

Pregnancy

Pregnancy in women with type 1 diabetes has been associated with adverse maternal and fetal outcomes. The incidence of spontaneous abortions, stillbirths, and congenital malformations in the offspring of diabetic mothers may be increased. Fortunately, these complications can be diminished by intensive glycemic regulation before and during pregnancy,[2] as shown in prospective as well as retrospective studies. Intensive glycemic regulation is now the standard of care for pregnancy and type 1 diabetes. In the DCCT, institution of intensive therapy in the preconception period or early during pregnancy was associated with rates of spontaneous abortion and congenital malformations similar to those in the nondiabetic population.[35]

Ideally, intensive management is started during the preconception period.[2] Clinical trials of stringent blood glucose control prior to and in the first trimester of pregnancy have demonstrated striking reductions in the rates of congenital malformations compared with diabetic women who did not participate in preconception care. The goal is to attain the lowest HbA1c level possible without the risk of severe hypoglycemia. HbA1c levels no greater than 1% above normal are desirable, and even lower levels are acceptable if tolerated without hypoglycemia. The management plan incorporates the integration of nutritional needs, self-monitoring of blood glucose, insulin administration, and an exercise plan, as previously described in the section on intensive glycemic management. The patient should be seen every 1–2 months during the preconception period to alter the management plan as needed and to obtain an optimal HbA1c level. Because retinopathy may accelerate during pregnancy, a comprehensive dilated eye examination should be done in the preconception period. In addition, baseline assessment of renal function by creatinine clearance and 24-hour urine albumin excretion are indicated, as are carefully obtained blood pressure measurements.

During the first trimester of pregnancy, insulin requirements may transiently decrease. This decrease may be related to a drop in nutrient intake from morning nausea or to a temporary increase in insulin sensitivity. Diabetic management during pregnancy should be shared by a diabetes team and an obstetric specialist, often with alternating visits at increasing intervals as the pregnancy progresses. Typically, insulin requirements gradually increase during pregnancy, especially in the third trimester when insulin-antagonist hormones are released by the maturing placenta. Management during and directly after delivery is the responsibility of the obstetric-anesthesia team. A drop in insulin requirements to the prepregnancy level is anticipated and is usually managed by intravenous fluids and decreasing doses of short-acting insulin. With these techniques, fetal morbidity and mortality rates are the same as in nondiabetic mothers.

Because pregnancy in type 1 diabetes may be associated with a worsening of diabetic retinopathy, increased ophthalmologic surveillance is indicated. In the DCCT, pregnant women who were previously in the conventional therapy group had a 2.48-fold greater risk of worsening of retinopathy compared with nonpregnant women.[34] The odds ratio peaked in the second trimester and persisted as long as 12 months after delivery. The long-term risk of progression of retinopathy, however, was not increased by pregnancy.

The effect of pregnancy on diabetic nephropathy was also studied in the DCCT,[34] which found a trend for an increase in albumin excretion rates during pregnancy. This effect was transient, and pregnancy had no long-term effect on the development of diabetic nephropathy. Other studies have shown that in type 1 diabetic women with normal albumin excretion rates or even with micro- or macroalbuminuria, pregnancy does not accelerate the course of nephropathy. In patients who already have evidence of renal insufficiency, pregnancy may accelerate nephropathy. Studies have shown that patients with creatinine clearance < 50 ml/min (or serum creatinine < 3 mg/dl) have about a 40% chance of worsening of renal function during pregnancy.

Key Points: Pregnancy

∽ Adverse fetal and maternal outcomes in pregnancy in type 1 diabetes are closely related to overall glycemic control.

∽ The complications of spontaneous abortions, stillbirths, and congenital malformations occur at rates similar to the nondiabetic population with intensive glycemic management (goal HbA1c ≤ 7%).

∽ Ideally, intensive management is started in the preconception period.

∽ Pregnant type 1 diabetic patients should be seen in alternate months (or more often) by the diabetes team and obstetric specialist.

∽ During the first trimester, there may be a decrease in insulin requirements. As pregnancy progresses (especially in the third trimester), an increase in insulin resistance, mediated by placental hormones, will increase insulin requirements.

∽ After delivery there is a drop in insulin requirements, which is best managed by intravenous fluids and insulin.

∽ A worsening of diabetic retinopathy may occur during pregnancy, and regular ophthalmologic surveillance is indicated. The risk is greater in patients on conventional therapy compared with those on intensive therapy.

∽ The long-term risk of progression of retinopathy or nephropathy is not altered by pregnancy.

References

1. Aiello LP, Gardner TW, King GL, et al: Diabetic retinopathy. Diabetes Care 21:143–156, 1998.
2. American Diabetes Association: Preconception care of women with diabetes. Diabetes Care 25:S82–S84, 2002.
3. American Diabetes Association: Standards of medical care for patients with diabetes mellitus. Diabetes Care 25:S33–S49, 2002.
4. American Diabetes Association: Treatment of hypertension in adults with diabetes. Diabetes Care 25:S71–S73, 2002.
5. Arauz-Pacheco C, Parrott MA, Raskin P: The treatment of hypertension in adult patients with diabetes. Diabetes Care 25:134–147, 2002.
6. Bakris GL, Williams M, Dworkin L, et al: Special Report: Preserving renal function in adults with hypertension and diabetes: A consensus approach. Am J Kidney Dis 36:646–661, 2000.
7. Bojestig M, Arnqvist HG, Hermansson G, et al: Declining incidence of nephropathy in insulin-dependent diabetes mellitus. N Engl J Med 330:15–18, 1994.
8. Brenner BM: Hemodynamically mediated glomerular injury and the progressive nature of kidney disease. Kidney Int 23:647–655, 1983.
9. Chaturvedi N, Sjølie A-K, Stephenson JM, et al: Effect of lisinopril on progression of retinopathy in normotensive people with type 1 diabetes. Lancet 351:28–31, 1998.
10. Crepaldi G, Carta Q, Deferrari G, et al: Effects of lisinopril and nifedipine on the

progression to overt albuminuria in IDDM patients with incipient nephropathy and normal blood pressure. The Italian Microalbuminuria Study Group in IDDM. Diabetes Care 21:104–110, 1998.

11. Gazis A, Page SR, Cockcroft JS: ACE inhibitors, diabetes and cardiovascular disease. Diabetologia 41:595–597, 1998.

12. Klein R: Hyperglycemia and microvascular and macrovascular disease in diabetes. Diabetes Care 18:258–268, 1995.

13. Klein R, Klein BEK, Moss SE, et al: The 10-year incidence of renal insufficiency in people with type 1 diabetes. Diabetes Care 22:743–751, 1999.

14. Knowles HCJ: Long term juvenile diabetes treated with unmeasured diet. Trans Assoc Am Physicians 84:95–101, 1971.

15. Krolewski AS, Warram JH, Christlieb AR, et al: The changing natural history of nephropathy in Type 1 diabetes. Am J Med 78:785–794, 1985.

16. Lewis E, Hunsicker L, Bain R, et al: The effect of angiotensin-converting-enzyme inhibition on diabetic nephropathy. N Engl J Med 329:1456–1462, 1993.

17. Lopes-Virella MF, Wohltmann HJ, Mayfield RK, et al: Effect of metabolic control on lipid, lipoprotein, and apolipoprotein levels in 55 insulin-dependent diabetic patients: A longitudinal study. Diabetes 32:20–25, 1983.

18. MacLeod JM, White KE, Tate H, et al: Efficient morphometric analysis of glomerular mesangium in insulin-dependent diabetic patients with early nephropathy. The European Study of the Progression of Renal Disease in type 1 (insulin dependent) Diabetes (ESPRIT) Study Group. Kidney Int 51:1624–1628, 1997.

19. Mathiesen ER, Hommel E, Hansen HP, et al: Randomised controlled trial of long term efficacy of captopril on preservation of kidney function in normotensive patients with insulin dependent diabetes and microalbuminuria. BMJ 319:24–25, 1999.

20. Mogensen CE: Microalbuminuria, blood pressure and diabetic renal disease: origin and development of ideas. Diabetologia 42:263–285, 1999.

21. Mogensen CE: Microalbuminuria predicts clinical proteinuria and early mortality in maturity onset diabetes. N Engl J Med 310:356–360, 1984.

22. Mogensen CE, Christensen CK: Predicting diabetic nephropathy in insulin-dependent patients. N Engl J Med 311:89–93, 1984.

23. Molitch ME: ACE inhibitors and diabetic nephropathy. Diabetes Care 17:756–760, 1994.

24. Østerby R, Gall M-A, Schmitz A: Glomerular structure and function in proteinuric Type 2 (non-insulin-dependent) diabetic patients. Diabetologia 36:1064–1070, 1993.

25. Parving HH: Renoprotection in diabetes: genetic and non-genetic risk factors and treatment. Diabetologia 41:745–759, 1998.

26. Parving HH, Chaturvedi N, Viberti GC, et al: Does microalbuminuria predict diabetic nephropathy? Diabetes 25:406–407, 2002.

27. Parving HH, Gall MA, Skøtt P, et al: Prevalence and causes of albuminuria in non-insulin-dependent diabetic patients. Kidney Int 41:758–762, 1992.

28. Pedersen MM, Schmitz A, Pedersen EB, et al: Acute and long-term renal effects of angiotensin converting enzyme inhibition in normotensive, normoalbuminuric insulin-dependent diabetic patients. Diabet Med 5:562–569, 1988.

29. Rudberg S, Osterby R, Bangstad HJ, et al: Effect of angiotensin converting enzyme inhibitor or beta blocker on glomerular structural changes in young microalbuminuric patients with type 1 (insulin-dependent) diabetes mellitus. Diabetologia 42:589–595, 1999.

30. The ACE Inhibitors in Diabetic Nephropathy Trialist Group: Should all patients with type 1 diabetes mellitus and microalbuminuria receive angiotensin-converting en-

zyme inhibitors? A meta-analysis of individual patient data. Ann Intern Med 134:370–379, 2001.

31. The Diabetes Control and Complications Trial/Epidemiology of Diabetes Interventions and Complications Research Group. Retinopathy and nephropathy in patients with type 1 diabetes four years after a trial of intensive therapy. N Engl J Med 342:381–389, 2000.

32. The Diabetes Control and Complications Trial Research Group: Early worsening of diabetic retinopathy in the diabetes control and complications trial. Arch Ophthalmol 116:874–886, 1998.

33. The Diabetes Control and Complications Trial (DCCT) Research Group: Effect of intensive diabetes management on macrovascular events and risk factors in the diabetes control and complications trial. Am J. Cardiol 75:894–903, 1995.

34. The Diabetes Control and Complications Trial Research Group: Effect of pregnancy on microvascular complications in the Diabetes Control and Complications Trial. Diabetes Care 23:1084–1091, 2000.

35. The Diabetes Control and Complications Trial Research Group: Pregnancy outcomes in the Diabetes Control and Complications Trial. Am J Obstet Gynecol 174:1343–1353, 1996.

36. The Diabetes Control and Complications Trial Research Group: The effect of intensive diabetes treatment on the progression of diabetic retinopathy in insulin-dependent diabetes mellitus. Arch Ophthalmol 113:36–51, 1995.

37. The Diabetes Control and Complications Trial Research Group: The effect of intensive treatment of diabetes on the development and progression of long-term complications in insulin-dependent diabetes mellitus. N Eng J Med 329:977–986, 1993.

38. The EUCLID Study Group: Randomised placebo-controlled trial of lisinopril in normotensive patients with insulin-dependent diabetes and normoalbuminuria or microalbuminuria. Lancet 349:1787–1792, 1997.

39. The European Study for the Prevention of Renal Disease in Type 1 Diabetes (ESPRIT) Study Group: Effect of 3 years of antihypertensive therapy on renal structure in type 1 diabetic patients with albuminuria. Diabetes 50:843–850, 2001.

40. Tuomilehto J, Borch-Johnson K, Molarius A, et al: Incidence of cardiovascular disease in type 1 (insulin-dependent) diabetic subjects with and without diabetic nephropathy in Finland. Diabetologia 41:784–790, 1998.

41. UK Prospective Diabetes Study Group: Efficacy of atenolol and captopril in reducing risk of macrovascular and microvascular complications in type 2 diabetes: UKPDS 39. BMJ 317:713–720, 1998.

42. UK Prospective Diabetes Study Group: Tight blood pressure control and risk of macrovascular and microvascular complications in type 2 diabetes: UKPDS 38. BMJ 317:703–713, 1998.

43. Viberti GC, Hill RD, Jarrett RJ: Microalbuminuria as a predictor of clinical nephropathy in insulin-dependent diabetes mellitus. Lancet i:1430–1432, 1982.

44. Viberti CB, Mogensen CE, Groop L, et al: Effect of captopril on progression to clinical proteinuria in patients with insulin-dependent diabetes mellitus and microalbuminuria. JAMA 271:275–279, 1994.

Type 1 Diabetes: Illustrative Cases

chapter

7

Uncomplicated Type 1 Diabetes with Prediabetic Phase and C-peptide Secretion

Type 1 diabetes has many faces. The following three cases illustrate that a period of altered glucose tolerance, asymptomatic hyperglycemia, or gestational diabetes may precede the appearance of type 1 diabetes. In one patient, reactive hypoglycemia was present for 2 years before the onset of type 1 diabetes.

Patient No. 1

A 42-year-old Caucasian woman reported that she had an elevated blood glucose transiently in 1980 and gestational diabetes (GDM) in 1995, which required 50 U of insulin daily. For 9 months after delivery, she was managed on diet alone but in 1996 was placed on insulin because of HbA1c of 7.1%. Pancreatic islet cell antibody tests were positive. Since then she has maintained HbA1c values in the range of 5.8–6.2%. Usual insulin doses are 5 U NPH before breakfast and 5 U NPH at bedtime with premeal lispro insulin, 1–3U. Her weight is steady at 60 kg; total insulin dose/24 hr = 0.33 U/kg. Blood pressure and lipid profile are normal. She has had fasting c-peptide levels of 0.6–0.8 ng/dl. She has no retinopathy and urine microalbumin levels are 5–7 mg/24 hours. She has hypothyroidism that is well controlled on 0.125 mg of L-thyroxine/day.

Comment. Type 1 diabetes may follow GDM, particularly in nonobese patients with positive islet antibodies. The presence of hypothyroidism is another clue to an autoimmune process in the thyroid and pancreas. This patient has maintained excellent glycemic control on low doses of insulin (0.33 U/kg), probably because of the presence of residual insulin secretion, as shown by fasting c-peptide levels of 0.6–0.8 ng/ml. Although laboratories may vary, we have found that a fasting level of < 1.0 ng/ml is consistent with type 1 diabetes, although higher levels are usually found in type 2 diabetes (Fig. 1). Experience has indicated that the patient may have a gradual loss of insulin secretion in the future. If so, her insulin

71

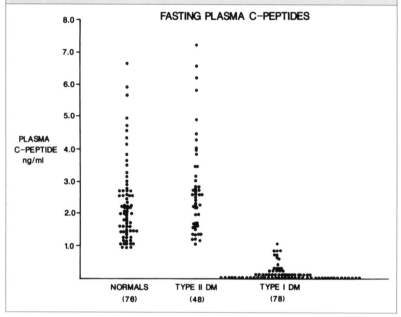

Figure 1. Plasma c-peptide levels after an overnight fast in nondiabetic individuals (n = 76), and people with type 2 (n = 48) or type 1 diabetes (n = 78). To convert ng/ml to pmol/ml, multiply by 0.331. (Unpublished data from author's research laboratory.)

requirements will rise and precise glycemic control will be more difficult. Bedtime insulin glargine with premeal lispro or aspart may be tried, or she may be placed on insulin pump therapy.

Patient No. 2

A 39-year-old nonobese Caucasian man was found to have a 3-hour postprandial plasma glucose of 187 mg/dl in 1993. An oral GTT yielded these values: F, 108; 1 hr, 225; 2 hr, 248; and 3 hr, 189 mg/dl. A second OGTT revealed comparable values. HbA1c was slightly elevated at 6.2%. He was placed on a meal plan with 50% carbohydrate, 30% fat, 20% protein, and 2200–2400 calories/day. He was very active; he ran 5 miles daily and had a black belt in Tae Kwon Do. After 9 months, his weight was constant, but HbA1c rose to 7.0%. He was placed on glyburide, 1.25 mg/day, with a fall in HbA1c to 5.2% after 6 months, followed by a subsequent rise to 8.5% at 12 months. He was switched to long-acting glipizide, 10 mg, plus metformin, 1.0 gm twice daily, and HbA1c fell to 7.2% at 6 months but rose to 9.6% at 1 year. He was then switched to insulin therapy, which (since 1996) has been 10–12 U NPH in the morning plus

10–12 U NPH at bedtime and premeal regular or lispro insulin at 3–5 U, adjusted for exercise. His HbA1c values over the 5 years range from 5.4% to 6.8%. His height is 6 feet, and his weight has been steady at 80 kg; total insulin requirement is about 0.5 U/kg. Recent (1998–2001) fasting c-peptide levels have been 0.7–0.9 ng/ml; nonfasting levels (taken in 1996) were 2.2–3.0 ng/ml. He has no retinopathy or microalbuminuria; blood pressure and plasma lipid values are normal. He has normal thyroid function, and islet cell antibody tests have been negative.

Comment. A diagnosis of diabetes was made by glucose tolerance testing, after a random nonfasting level was found to be high. He was successfully managed on diet and oral agents for over 2 years, but eventually his HbA1c was 9.6% on combined oral sulfonylurea and metformin therapy. He was slim and quite active, with excellent physical conditioning, indicating insulin sensitivity. Although nonobese type 2 diabetes cannot be completely ruled out, it is more likely that he has slowly evolving type 1 diabetes. Despite excellent glycemic control, fasting plasma c-peptide levels are now below 1ng/ml (Fig. 1), and he requires split doses of insulin, plus premeal lispro insulin, for excellent diabetic control. He has a low insulin requirement of 0.5 U/kg of exogenous insulin, supplemented by endogenous insulin secretion. There is no evidence of microvascular complications of eyes or kidneys, and the progression of these problems should be markedly slowed by intensive therapy. In the future, a switch to bedtime doses of glargine insulin plus premeal lispro or aspart insulin will be considered, particularly if hypoglycemia becomes a problem. Insulin pump therapy is another excellent option for the future.

As noted, the patient is very active physically. He has learned to cut his NPH dose in the morning by up to 50% and to drop the bedtime dose if glucose values are below 100 mg/dl after a day of exercise. He also carries carbohydrate supplements, particularly with long-distance running. Severe hypoglycemia has not been an issue to date.

Patient No. 3

A 30-year-old Caucasian woman was first seen because of reactive hypoglycemia, as documented by OGTT on two occasions (in 1990 and 1992) when 2-hour values fell below 50 mg/dl with symptoms. The OGTTs were otherwise within normal limits.

In 1994, she presented to her primary care physician with a random plasma glucose of 427 mg/dl and HbA1c of 10.8%. She had a history of 2 weeks of increasing polydipsia, polyuria, and weight loss. She was not ketotic. She responded quickly to insulin therapy and was maintained on low doses of NPH in the morning and at bedtime with premeal regular insulin until she was switched to insulin pump in 1996. Total insulin dose is 24–26 units; her weight is 54 kg (dose = 0.46 U/kg). She has had fasting c-peptide levels as follows (1994–1997): 1.1, 0.8, and 0.6 ng/ml. With a nutrient stimulus, these levels have risen to 3.2, 1.4 ng/ml. She has positive islet antibodies and normal thyroid function. There is no retinopathy or microalbuminuria. Blood pressure and lipid values are normal.

Comment. This is an unusual story of reactive hypoglycemia before the sudden onset of type 1 diabetes. Older studies have indicated that reactive hypoglycemia, usually 3–5 hours after an oral glucose load, may precede the diagnosis of type 2 diabetes. Such patients often have a 3-hour GTT in the diabetic or IGT range, which precedes the late dip of plasma glucose below 50mg/dl. This patient did not have such a curve but did have symptomatic reactive hypoglycemia 2 hours after the glucose was ingested. It is likely that this issue, which is quite common in young women, is not connected to the subsequent appearance of type 1 diabetes.

Like patients 1 and 2, this patient maintained insulin secretory ability for up to 4 years after the diagnosis and intensive treatment of type 1 diabetes. Serial values over a 3-year period showed a gradual decrease in fasting and stimulated levels. Her insulin requirements have remained low, well below the 0.6–0.7 U/kg required in the intensive management cohort in the DCCT. Hopefully, long-term intensive management in all three of these patients will preserve beta cell function. If so, as shown in the DCCT, these patients will have fewer hypoglycemic reactions and slower progression (or even long-term prevention) of microvascular complications. These three patients illustrate the importance of vigorous intensive glycemic management very early in the course of type 1 diabetes.

Type 1 Diabetes with Microvascular Disease

Patient No. 4

A 51-year-old Caucasian woman was followed regularly for 20 years. Type 1 diabetes had a symptomatic onset in 1972, and she was placed on insulin therapy. For the first 15 years, she was managed on equal doses of ultralente insulin before breakfast and supper, with total daily dosage of 18–20 U. This was supplemented with 15–18 U of regular insulin, usually 5–6 U, 30 minutes before each of three daily meals. Her food habits were regular, and she ran 3–4 miles at least 3 times weekly. On these days, she would cut the ultralente insulin by 10–20%, and avoided severe hypoglycemia. HbA1c values were in the 4.3–6.8% range 90% of the time, and there was an occasional value of 7–8%. Weight was stable at about 52 kg; insulin requirements were approximately 0.70 U/kg. She had two successful pregnancies.

For the past 5 years, she has been on insulin pump therapy, with basal rate of 0.8 U/hr and premeal doses of lispro prescribed at 4–6 U. Although this schedule approximated her previous 0.70 U/kg requirement, HbA1c values are consistently higher and are usually in the 7.7–8.9% range. Weight is unchanged. She has minimal background retinopathy, 5–7 mg albumin in the urine/24 hours, normal blood pressure and lipid profiles. Repeated fasting c-peptide levels, and islet antibodies have been undetectable. She has no thyroid disease.

Comment. The patient's course is instructive in several ways. In spite of 20 years of type 1 diabetes, with no residual insulin secretion, she avoided severe hypoglycemia and maintained HbA1c levels at the target of ≤7% for the first 15 years. She has only minimal background retinopathy, no microalbuminuria, and no neuropathy. This finding is comparable to results in DCCT in the group of patients who were intensively managed over a shorter average period of 6.2 years.

In the past 5 years, however, there has been a lapse from this intensive control, and HbA1c values are generally 1–2% higher than in the first 15 years despite insulin pump therapy, with a schedule of relatively constant insulin doses and controlled weight and diet. The DCCT demonstrated that a period of tight glycemic control continued to decrease the progression of retinopathy, even after 4 years of less stringent control. The same phenomenon may be operative in this patient. The progression of retinopathy is related not only to the absolute HbA1c value but also to many years of exposure to hyperglycemia. We suspect that this patient will begin to show progression of retinopathy and, perhaps, appearance of microalbuminuria, if suboptimal diabetic control continues. Of course, we have counseled her many times and have prescribed numerous changes in her management schedule. She admits she used the basal infusion rate on most occasions and chose not to take the prescribed premeal lispro doses for fear of hypoglycemia and weight gain. It is not completely clear why she is less vigilant about intensive management recently, but several life stresses appear to be involved.

A promising aspect is that she never has smoked cigarettes and has BP of 100/60 mmHg. Since only about 30% of type 1 patients get diabetic nephropathy, she may be protected against this complication despite a rising HbA1c—probably for genetic reasons.

Patient No. 5

A 30-year-old Caucasian woman has had type 1 diabetes since the age of 15. She was first seen about 6 years ago because of two episodes of severe early-morning hypoglycemia in the past year, requiring treatment in the emergency department. She had been taking 13 U NPH before breakfast and before supper, supplemented with 6–8 U of regular insulin before each of three meals. She had a normal weight of 62 kg;

insulin dosage was about 0.76 U/kg. She is a vegetarian and exercises by jogging 3–4 miles daily from 6–8 p.m. Fasting c-peptide level is unmeasurable.

We believed that the severe reactions were due to the presupper NPH and regular insulin acting at 2–3 a.m., exacerbated by increased insulin sensitivity from the postsupper exercise. We switched her to a regimen of 9–10 U ultralente before breakfast and supper and added lispro insulin in doses of 5–8 U before meals. This regimen provided about 0.65 U/kg, as a basal insulin with smaller, delayed peaking compared with NPH. She adjusted the ultralente and supper lispro insulin doses down by 1–3 U according to exercise planning and assessment of blood glucose responses to exercise. We followed her for 5 years, and the majority of HbA1c values were in the 5–6% range, with occasional mild, but no severe, hypoglycemia. She had no retinopathy or microalbuminuria; BP was 90–100/50–60 mmHg; and lipids and thyroid function were normal.

In late December, 2000, she became pregnant with her first child. Excellent diabetic control continued, and insulin requirements doubled by August, 2001. At this time (36 weeks) she had gained 16 kg and had 3+ pitting edema. Blood pressure was 102/62 mmHg, but a 24-hour urine collection revealed 567 mg of total protein. There was no retinopathy. She was kept at bed rest, diuresed 5 kg, and delivered a normal 8-lb, 2-oz infant at 39 weeks. Her insulin requirements fell to the preconception levels. We saw her one month after delivery. She was 1 kg above preconception weight, and BP was 104/70 mmHg. She had no edema, and spot urine showed 2 mg of albumin/gm creatinine (normal).

Comment. This patient has had extremely well controlled type 1 diabetes for 15 years. She has no retinopathy or neuropathy but has had severe hypoglycemic reactions. Late in pregnancy, she developed edema and proteinuria, which quickly cleared after delivery. She maintains excellent glycemic control on the expected insulin requirement of 0.6–0.7 U/kg.

Her long-term prognosis is excellent. The transient proteinuria and edema late in pregnancy were of great concern at the time. However, it was not accompanied by hypertension, and it quickly cleared after delivery. Proteinuria during pregnancy does not necessarily predict diabetic nephropathy. Although the mechanism is not clearly understood, we believe that she will continue to show normal renal function with no or minimal retinopathy for many years to come. Of interest, she tried insulin pump therapy for a short time but decided to go back to multiple-dose insulin therapy. Although this has not been our general experience, it illustrates that insulin therapy must be tailored for each individual patient.

Patient No. 6

A 44-year-old type 1 diabetic man was first seen in 1994. Diabetes was diagnosed first at the age of 13, with the typical symptoms, hospitalization, and immediate insulin therapy. He was managed on a single dose of 40–45 U NPH each morning until 1994, when he was switched to 14 U ultralente and 7–8 U regular insulin before breakfast and supper. He has had several episodes of severe hypoglycemia and, when first seen, had background retinopathy, numbness of both feet, and impotence for 3 months. He did not smoke. He has a history of heart attacks and strokes on his mother's side. Physical exam: BP 110/82 mm Hg diminished-to-absent pinprick sensation over toes and soles of both feet, absent ankle jerks.

Diabetic management was 26–30 U (70/30) in the morning and 24U NPH (at bedtime), with 8–12 U regular or lispro before supper. In 2001, he was switched to insulin glargine, 30 U at bedtime, plus premeal lispro, 6–12 U, with a fall in HbA1c to < 7%.

LDL-C was consistently over 100 mg/dl and fell to 84 mg/dl after atorvastatin, 10 mg/day, was started. Blood pressure was usually above 130/80 mmHg and responded to lisinopril, 10 mg, plus amlodipine, 5 mg/day. Viagra, up to 100 mg/day, was prescribed with some success. He developed the rare complication of a Charcot joint after fracturing his right first toe.

Comment. The patient had one dose of NPH prescribed for the first 21 years of his type 1 diabetes. It is impossible to provide adequate insulin therapy for type 1 diabetes with a single dose of any type of insulin. At the very least, two doses are always needed for 24-hour coverage, and three to four doses are needed for intensive management. When first seen in 1995, his HbA1c was 9.6% and probably was reflective of his long-term control. He had background retinopathy which progressed to

| | | | | | | | Urine | |
Date	BP	HbA1c	Chol	Trig	HDL-C	LDL-C	Microalb/Cr	Retinopathy
8/95	110/82	9.6%	202	63	43	146	Normal	Background
10/98	140/90	8.3%	210	87	45	148		Background Vitreous Hemorrhage (laser)
10/00	132/86	8.1%	152	81	52	84	Normal	Proliferative DR Laser treatment
9/01	126/80	7.7%						
2/02	131/80	6.8%						Charcot joint

| Laboratory Values |
| DR = diabetic retinopathy. |

vitreous hemorrhage and proliferative retinopathy that required laser therapy and vitrectomy. He also has suffered from peripheral sensory neuropathy and impotence but has had no microalbuminuria.

Two other issues increase his cardiovascular risk. First, his plasma lipid profile was borderline to elevated before atorvastatin therapy was started. There was an immediate fall in cholesterol to 152 mg/dl, a rise in HDL-C to 52 mg/dl, and a fall in LDL-C to 84 mg/dl. This therapy is expected to be cardioprotective despite his high risk. Blood pressures were low initially but frequently exceeded the recommended goal of < 130/80 mmHg. It took a combination of ACE inhibitor and calcium channel blocker therapy to drop BP to acceptable levels. This therapy also should be cardioprotective, as should the regimen of 81 mg of enteric-coated aspirin daily.

Glycemic control has not been optimal. A recent switch to insulin glargine and premeal lispro insulin appears to be providing the 24-hour basal and bolus insulin schedule needed for more acceptable HbA1c levels.

Viagra has helped the erectile dysfunction, but he has developed a Charcot joint in his right foot. This complication is related to his long-standing peripheral and autonomic neuropathy and was not prevented by improved glycemic control.

This patient illustrates some of the many difficulties inherent in a long period of inadequate glycemic regulation. Our current goals are to improve glycemic management and also to provide optimal cardioprotective management to prevent potentially lethal cardiovascular complications. Thus, in longstanding type 1 diabetes with complications, the emphasis may change from preventing microvascular to preventing macrovascular complications. He wears a non–weight-bearing cast on the right calf and foot to avoid further breakdown of the Charcot Joint.

Type 1 Diabetes with Advanced Complications

Patient No. 7

A 54-year-old Caucasian man, a pediatric endocrinologist, had the sudden onset of type 1 diabetes at the age of 15. He was started on 40 U of lente insulin daily and stayed on approximately the same dose until he was first seen by our group at the age of 46. He was self-referred and was concerned about recurrent nocturnal hypoglycemic reactions and the need for laser therapy in both eyes over the past 3 years. He had a 10-year history of slowly progressive multiple sclerosis manifested primarily by leg weakness, which had apparently stabilized with interferon therapy administered by his neurologist.

His physical examination was negative except for extensor muscle weakness of both thighs and peripheral sensory neuropathy. BP was 126/76 mmHg, and retinal examination showed laser scars bilaterally. His weight was 139 lb (ideal weight-150–160 lb).

His insulin schedule was changed to 30–35 U of 70/30 insulin before breakfast and 10U NPH at bedtime. He refused to do glucose monitoring but would take 6–8 U of lispro before a large supper several times a week. He gained weight to 157 lb (71.3 kg). Glycemic control was markedly improved, and he had one early-morning insulin reaction. When elevated cholesterol and LDL-C were noted in 1993–1994, he was first placed on simvastatin, then switched to atorvastatin, 10 mg/day, in 1997. Except for a persistently low HDL-C, lipid profile has improved markedly. In 1994, modest elevation of systolic BP was noted, and microalbuminuria increased. He was placed on monopril, 20 mg/day, and had a fall in urinary albumin and in BP on this regimen. His newly discovered hypothyroidism responded well to L-thyroxine, 125 mg/day. Renal function, as estimated by creatinine clearance, has been stable at 116–133 mg/min. His retinopathy has not progressed, and multiple sclerosis is stable.

Comment. This is another type 1 diabetic patient who was inadequately treated on 1 dose of intermediate insulin for 31 years despite the fact that he is a pediatric endocrinologist! He was seen by our group at the time of completion and reporting of the DCCT results. He already had proliferative retinopathy, microalbuminuria, slight BP elevation, and an atherogenic lipid profile. He was also found to be mildly hypothyroid. On a combination of split-dose insulin at an intensive management dosage of 0.63 U/kg, he gained to his ideal weight of 155 lb and maintained HbA1c in the 7–8% range without severe hypoglycemia (without SMBG testing). Lipid profile was characteristic of uncontrolled type 1 diabetes and diabetic nephropathy. He needed statin therapy in addition to better glycemic control for optimal management. The per-

			Chol	Trig	HDL-C	LDL-C		mg/24hr		
Date	BP	HbA1c	mg/dl	mg/dl	mg/dl	mg/dl	Cr	Ur Alb	TSH	FT4
1993	126/26	11%	194	112	25	147	1.0	255	11.4	1.0
1994	144/86	7.9%	208	59	28	168	0.9	792	2.4	1.4
1995	120/70	7.9%	165	125	20	125	1.0	417	—	—
1996	150/80	7.5%	—	—	—	—	1.0	356		
1997	130/60	8.1%	180	150	24	126	1.0	179	0.93	01.3
1998	130/74	7.8%	116	160	21	63	1.0	320		
2000	120/60	7.0%	116	171	26	56	1.1	163		
2001	120/70	7.1%	117	94	26	72	1.1	394	0.88	1.0

Serial Laboratory Values

sistently low HDL-C is unusual in insulin-treated type 1 diabetic patients with good glycemic control and statin therapy. Fibrate therapy may be started, with monitoring of liver function and creatinine kinase values.

His nephropathy has not progressed since glycemic control was improved and ACE inhibitor therapy was used. Before the recognition of the importance of these two strategies to prevent progression of nephropathy, it is likely that he would have progressed to renal failure over the 8 years during which we have followed him. Mild hypothyroidism is an indication of autoimmune disease. The combination of multiple sclerosis, type 1 diabetes, and hypothyroidism is rare but suggests an autoimmune basis for his neurologic disease. Finally, because of his high cardiovascular risk, he is maintained on 81 mg of enteric-coated aspirin daily.

Patient No. 8

A 39-year-old Caucasian man has had type 1 diabetes since age 3 years. When first seen in 1993, he had been on one dose of 22 U NPH + 12 U regular before breakfast daily for about 8–10 years and had been on single morning doses for over 90% of his diabetic life. He had recently married, and his wife urged him to seek improved diabetic care. He did no SMBG monitoring and had frequent prelunch insulin reactions as well as a history of several admissions in the past 10 years for diabetic ketoacidosis. He was recently referred to a retinal specialist by an ophthalmologist but had not had laser therapy. History was otherwise negative except that he was a cigarette smoker (1–1½ packs/day as an adult). Physical examination revealed an underweight man (139 lb, height 70 inches) with BP of 110/80 mmHg and nonproliferative diabetic neuropathy.

He was initially managed on 16U NPH+5U Regular in the morning and 18U NPH at bedtime, with presupper doses of 3–7 U regular insulin. After a few years, he was switched to ultralente insulin, 16–18 U before breakfast and supper, with 4–8 U lispro before meals. He gained

Serial Laboratory Values										
Date	BP	HbA1c	Chol mg/dl.	Trig. mg/dl	HDL-C mg/dl	LDL-C mg/dl	Cr.	mg/24hr Ur. Alb.	TSH	FT4
1993	110/80	10.4%					0.7	328		
1994	120/80	6.7%					0.9	223		
1996	110/70	6.6%	177	83	34	126	0.9	137	1.54	7.4
1997	118/80	6.9%	174	47	29	136	0.8	29	0.81	
1998	120/80	6.7%	183	35	54	114	0.8	42		
1999	90/60	7.3%	200	68	52	134	0.9	22		
2001	116/68	7.1%	131	84	52	62	0.9	16		

from 139 to 160 lb (73 kg). His average total insulin dosage is 50 U/day (0.68 U/kg). This is a typical intensive management dosage. Glycemic regulation has been good except for hypoglycemia when HbA1c was below 7%.

In 1993, when we first saw him after many years of poor diabetic control on single morning insulin doses, he had HbA1c of 10.4%, progressive retinopathy, and elevated urinary albumin excretion. He required laser therapy in 1994, but retinopathy has been stable since then. This complication may have represented transient worsening with intensification of glycemic control in 1993. The albuminuria has fallen to normal 24 hour levels, with very good glycemic control and lisinopril, 10 mg daily. This dose was cut to 5 mg in 1999 because of symptoms of postural hypotension, but urinary albumin remains normal on the lower dosage. In 1999, after his lipid profile worsened as HbA1c rose, he was placed on atorvastatin, 10 mg/day, with an excellent response, as demonstrated by low cholesterol and LDL-C levels.

He has gone through several different smoking cessation programs, including nicotine patch, hypnosis, and bupropion therapy, but has not been able to completely stop smoking cigarettes for a long period. He currently smokes ½–1 pack/day and was referred to a smoking cessation program. He takes 81 mg of enteric-coated aspirin daily.

This patient is an example of the effects of long-term inadequate glycemic control (plus smoking) on the microcirculation of the retinas and renal glomeruli. If not treated aggressively from 1993 onward with glycemic regulation and ACE inhibitor therapy, he would have had progressive diabetic nephropathy leading to renal failure as well as more frequent laser therapy for proliferative diabetic retinopathy and/or maculopathy. Hyperlipoproteinemia is often associated with maculopathy, and it is likely that statin therapy is helpful.

Patient No. 9

A 52-year-old Caucasian man was diagnosed with type 1 diabetes in 1968 at the age of 19 years. He had typical symptoms and a 10-lb weight loss. After a 6-month trial of oral agents, he was switched to a combination of NPH and regular insulin in doses of 30–40 U before breakfast. For about 10 years, he was managed on 10 U of ultralente at bedtime with premeal regular insulin doses of 3–5 U.

In 1985, he was evaluated at Johns Hopkins for the DCCT, but retinopathy was too advanced, and he was enrolled instead in the Early Treatment Diabetic Retinopathy Study (ETDRS), in which he received laser therapy for proliferative diabetic retinopathy. He was found to be hypertensive and was placed on enalapril, 10 mg/day; diltiazem, 240 mg/day; and furosemide, 10 mg/day. He has had impotence for about

5 years and is also aware that kidney function has been abnormal for 8–10 years.

We first saw him in 1996, and physical examination showed that he was normotensive (BP of 120/78 mmHg with no postural drop), with bilateral laser scars, good peripheral pulses, absent sensation over soles of feet, and diminished ankle jerk reflexes.

He was started on 9–10 units of ultralente insulin before breakfast and supper and took 3–6 U lispro at each meal. His weight was 105 kg and total dosage was approximately 0.25U/kg. HbA1c responded well, and he had few hypoglycemic episodes.

He was jointly followed by a nephrologist, and antihypertensive therapy was adjusted to maintain BP <130/80 mmHg whenever possible, using a combination of ACE inhibitor and ARB therapies as well as a calcium channel blocker and diuretic therapy. Serum creatinine and creatinine clearance have remained stable over a 4-year period. In 1999, because of an LDL-C value that was consistently over 100 mg/dl, 10 mg of atorvastatin was started. LDL-C fell to 80 mg/dl. He was found to have an elevated plasma homocysteine level of 23.5 in 1996 (top normal; 12 μmol/L). With folic acid (7 mg/day), vitamin B_6 (50 mg/day) and vitamin B_{12} (1000 mcg/day) therapy, there was a fall toward normal. Folic acid will be raised and vitamins B_6 (50 mg) and B_{12} (1 mg) will be added daily, with a goal of plasma homocysteine level < 12 μmol/L.

Comment. Several important points are illustrated by this patient's course. First, after about 17 years of standard diabetic management, he was found to have preproliferative retinopathy and required laser therapy in the ETDRS. He had hypertension and probably also had diabetic renal disease at the time. He was started on ACE inhibitor and calcium channel blocker therapy in 1985, when both classes of agents were newly approved by the FDA and collaborative trials of their use in diabetic patients with nephropathy and hypertension were not available. In any case, it is likely that aggressive antihypertensive and ACE inhibitor therapy has kept renal insufficiency from progressing over the past 15 years. Because of a recent increase in urinary albumin excretion, further adjustment of these drugs may be needed. One experimental idea has been to add an ARB to

									mg/24 hr	Plasma
			Chol.	Trig	HDL-C	LDL-C				
Date	BP	HbA1c	mg/dl.	mg/dl	mg/dl	mg/dl	Cr	Cr Cl	Ur Alb	Homocysteine
1996	120/78	8.1%	194	127	39	130	2.5	54	144	23.5
1998	110/60	7.5%	166	117	38	105	2.3	57	261	
1991	140/72	6.9%	173	105	37	115	2.5	66		16.2
2000	130/70	6.6%	144	81	48	80	2.6	53	442	16

Serial Laboratory Values

ACE inhibitor therapy, because there are sources of angiotensin II not produced by converting enzyme action on angiotensin I.

A second issue is the presence of high plasma homocysteine levels, which often are seen in renal failure of any cause. Many reports have described this phenomenon in diabetic patients, even with modest elevations of serum creatinine. In one study, 35% of type 1 diabetics with disease of at least 10 years' duration had elevated plasma homocysteine levels. Homocysteine is a predictor of cardiovascular disease, and the risk rises with levels above 12–13 µmol/L. Folic acid increases the metabolism of homocysteine, and plasma levels fall with adequate doses. In the presence of renal insufficiency, high doses (up to 10 mg/day) may be needed. Vitamins B_6 and B_{12} act as cofactors to help normalize the abnormal methionine–homocysteine metabolism that may be present.

Many physicians now use vitamin therapy in patients with high plasma homocysteine levels. Controlled clinical trials are under way, with the postulate that returning homocysteine levels to normal will delay or prevent the occurrence of cardiovascular events without undue risk. Evidence of this type is needed before this approach becomes a standard of care.

Summary of Cases of Type 1 Diabetes

The nine cases presented above illustrate the diverse nature of type 1 diabetes. If the disease is recognized and treated aggressively at an early stage, some insulin secretion may be maintained for years. Diabetic management is simplified, and microvascular complications proceed at a very slow rate. On the other hand, with standard insulin management (one daily dose of intermediate insulin), the appearance of complications of the eyes, kidneys, and nerves usually is accelerated. Intensive management at this stage, however, with basal insulin and premeal short-acting insulin can still delay progression of retinopathy, nephropathy, and neuropathy. In patients who are destined to have diabetic renal disease, which is recognized by microalbuminuria and rising blood pressure, ACE inhibitor therapy, along with intensive glucose management, can arrest progression of nephropathy to renal failure. Even in the presence of early renal failure, these measures protect against further deterioration of renal function.

Patients who develop diabetic nephropathy often have associated cardiovascular risk factors that must be aggressively treated. Examples include hypertension, dyslipidemia, and elevated plasma homocysteine levels. Generally combinations of two or more agents for each of these issues, along with low doses (81 mg) of enteric-coated aspirin, are indicated as cardioprotective agents.

The policy for our team in the intensive management program has been to keep track of all of this information with a simple flow sheet. A reminder system of this nature, with serial values entered over the years, is an invaluable addition to successful long-term diabetic management. At present, computerized systems are available or under development to accomplish the same ends as the serial written record. Whichever system is used (or both), it is critical for long-term care to follow key objective parameters and to observe response to therapy with appropriate goals established.

Type 2 Diabetes

chapter
8

Pathophysiology

Insulin resistance and diminished pancreatic insulin secretion combine to produce type 2 diabetes mellitus.[43,44,61,62] Debate continues as to which is the primary defect.[45] Longitudinal studies in certain populations, such as Pima Indians and Mexican Americans, suggest that insulin resistance may be the initial, predominant lesion.[31] In other populations, such as white Europeans, insulin deficiency may be the primary defect.[42] Both insulin resistance and diminished insulin release are seen in low-birth-weight infants, and birth weight is inversely correlated with the risk of type 2 diabetes in adults.[47] Type 2 diabetes is a heterogeneous disorder, and the earliest defect may be insulin resistance in some patients and deficient insulin secretion in others.

In any case, it is generally accepted that both defects coexist in most people with type 2 diabetes. Before the stage of fasting hyperglycemia, patients progress from normal to impaired glucose tolerance. In the presence of insulin resistance, which is usually associated with overweight (or obesity) and a sedentary lifestyle, the pancreas of a person destined to progress to type 2 diabetes loses its ability to secrete insulin immediately after a glucose stimulus. This decrease in first-phase insulin secretion results in a higher than normal postprandial glucose rise. This, in turn, stimulates the pancreas to secrete an abundance of second-phase insulin and, in spite of insulin resistance, plasma glucose returns almost to normal. As shown in Yalow and Berson's first classic studies in overweight type 2 diabetics,[60] there is a lag in early insulin secretion, followed by relative hyperinsulinemia in the presence of elevated plasma glucose levels. Subsequent investigators argued that the insulin responses, although greater than in controls, were less than would be expected if the control subjects had comparable hyperglycemia. Furthermore, obesity and insulin resistance contributed to the apparent hyperinsulinemia.

By the time fasting hyperglycemia is seen, the pancreas has already lost 50–60% of its secretory capacity, and it is clear that insulin deficiency is a major contributor to the fasting hyperglycemia of type 2 diabetes. Increasing duration of type 2 diabetes leads to further loss of beta cell function (Fig. 1). At fasting plasma glucose levels of 200 mg/dl or greater, the

Figure 1. Pancreatic beta cell function in the UKPDS over a 6-year period. Panel *A*, Results from 376 type 2 patients allocated to diet (*open circles*) and 51 allocated to sulfonylurea therapy (*solid triangles*). Panel B, Results from a subset of 110 patients allocated to diet (*open circles*) compared with 159 patients allocated to metformin (*crosses*) and those allocated to sulfonylurea therapy (*solid triangles*). (From UKPDS. Diabetes 44:1249–1258, 1995, with permission.)

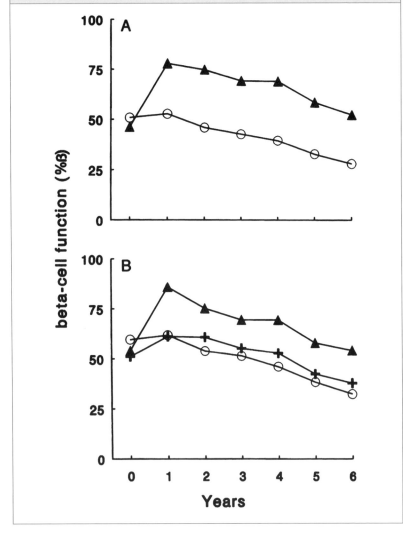

pancreas of the type 2 diabetic secretes only a low amount of basal insulin that is inadequate to control post-meal hyperglycemia. Fasting and postprandial glucose levels are greatly in excess of levels in nondiabetics. At plasma glucose levels of about 140 mg/dl and higher, the output of glucose by the liver increases. The fasting plasma glucose increases in direct proportion to the hepatic glucose output, which accounts for the overnight fasting hyperglycemia that is diagnostic of diabetes.[13]

Concomitant with progressive insulin deficiency is resistance to insulin's action to promote glucose uptake by insulin-responsive tissues as well as resistance by the liver to the action of insulin to suppress hepatic glucose production. Plasma free fatty acid levels are elevated, reflecting insulin resistance by adipose tissue. To make matters worse, prolonged hyperglycemia accentuates the insulin resistance; thus, what little insulin is present is relatively ineffective in lowering plasma glucose.

These pathophysiologic components underlie the recommendations for therapy in people with type 2 diabetes (Table 1). Insulin resistance can be reduced by modest weight reduction, exercise and physical conditioning, and drugs of the insulin-sensitizing group: thiazolidinediones and metformin. Furthermore, any therapy (such as insulin) that returns elevated plasma glucose levels to normal will remove the component of insulin resistance due to glucose toxicity and thereby improves insulin sensitivity. The first-phase insulin secretion may be stimulated, particularly in patients with pancreatic reserves that are not profoundly depleted, by drugs of the meglitinide class. In patients with very depleted beta cell reserve (i.e., type 2 diabetes with persistent fasting plasma glucose levels over 250 mg/dl), one can mimic the depleted first-phase insulin response with rapid-acting insulin analogs, lispro or aspart. Basal insulin supply may be augmented by sulfonylurea drugs or intermediate- to long-acting

Table 1. Treatment Strategies for People with Type 2 Diabetes	
Target	**Strategy**
Insulin resistance	Weight reduction
	Exercise
	Metformin
	Thiazolidinediones
	Normoglycemia (glucose toxicity)
First-phase insulin release	Meglitinides
	Short-acting sulfonylurea
	Lispro or aspart insulin
Late-phase or basal insulin release	Long-acting sulfonylureas
	Intermediate- and long-acting insulin
Dietary carbohydrate	
Postprandial glycemia	Acarbose, miglitol

insulin preparations. Finally, combinations of basal and first-phase insulin therapeutic strategies may be used. Each of these approaches is considered further in the chapters on treatment of type 2 diabetes. A perspective on management of type 2 diabetes derived from the pathophysiology of the disease is given in Fig. 2.

Natural History of Type 2 Diabetes

As noted in the consideration of its pathophysiology, type 2 diabetes is a progressive disease. Various stages in the disorder are shown in Figure 2. A genetic susceptibility has been demonstrated in family studies, particularly in studies of nondiabetic identical twins of parents with type 2 diabetes. The ultimate risk of the nondiabetic identical twin for developing type 2 diabetes ranges from 60% to 90%. Precise genetic markers are not available; the disorder is polygenic, and defects in a variety of

Figure 2. Type 2 diabetes is viewed in four stages, usually characterized by increasing duration and progressive elevation of plasma glucose profiles. Insulin resistance increases from glucose toxicity, as first- and second-phase insulin secretion is diminished over time, and hepatic glucose output increases. Therapeutic strategies are defined that address key defects at each stage of type 2 diabetes.

A perspective on management of type 2 diabetes.

TYPE 2 D.M.

STAGE	I	II	III	IV
USUAL DURATION	0	5	10	> 10 YR.
PLASMA GLUCOSE	IGT	126 - 150	151 - 200	> 200 mg/dl (FPG)

PATHO PHYSIOLOGY

INSULIN RESISTANCE	PRESENT + INCREASES (GLUCOSE TOXICITY)			
1st PHASE INS. SECR.	↓	↓↓	↓↓↓	0
BASAL INS. SECR.	↑	→	↓	↓↓
HEP. GLUC. OUTPUT	NL	↑	↑↑	↑↑↑

DRUG THERAPY

METFORMIN, TZD: CONSIDER AT ALL STAGES (I - IV)

SU/MEGLITINIDE: MOST EFFECTIVE FPG 126 - 200 (II, III)

BASAL INSULIN: START AT STAGE III, CONTINUE IV

BOLUS INSULIN: START AT STAGE IV, CONSIDER EARLIER

tissues, including the pancreas, muscle, and other tissues, are under study. It is critical, however, in the absence of a genetic marker, that first-degree relatives of people with type 2 diabetes be aware that they are at high risk for the disease and that glucose testing is recommended. Furthermore, members of populations with high prevalence rates (American Indians, African or Hispanic Americans, Pacific Islanders, Asian Americans) are also at high risk, most likely for genetic reasons.

Environmental influences clearly play a role. As the incidence of overweight and obesity increase in the United States, so does the incidence of type 2 diabetes. Physical inactivity, caloric excess, and lack of physical conditioning are important. Impairment of glucose tolerance or diabetes is now seen with increasing frequency in people under the age of 20, an age group in which type 1 diabetes had previously accounted for the majority of cases. One study found that for every 500-kcal increase in daily energy expenditure, the age-adjusted risk for type 2 diabetes was reduced by 6%.[27] This reduction is mediated by an increase in insulin sensitivity, not by weight reduction. A recent study in Finland[59] and the Diabetes Prevention Program[14] showed that the risk of progression from impaired glucose tolerance to fasting hyperglycemia is reduced 58% by vigorous lifestyle changes in diet and exercise.

During this phase before the development of IGT and/or type 2 diabetes, there is often a constellation of findings that contribute to an increased vascular risk. First termed *syndrome X* by G. Reaven,[46] the syndrome has been expanded in its definition and has been variously called *insulin resistance syndrome* or *metabolic syndrome.* Its components may be present in various combinations and include centripetal obesity, insulin resistance, glucose intolerance, dyslipidemia, hyperinsulinemia, microalbuminuria, hypertension, and a prothrombotic state with elevated plasma levels of plasminogen activator inhibitor (PAI-I). The prevalence of the syndrome in the U.S. in the Third National Health and Nutrition Survey (NHANES III, 1988–1994) was 24% overall and reached 43% in people > 60 years of age.[19] Thus, it is now clear that a number of cardiovascular risk factors may be present in a substantial proportion of the U.S. population before the diagnosis of IGT or type 2 diabetes and that these risk factors undoubtedly contribute to the accelerated atherosclerosis that is typical of the disease. Approaches to diagnosis and therapy of the metabolic syndrome and the evidence in support of these approaches are discussed in Chapter 10.

Although the majority of people with IGT eventually progress to fasting hyperglycemia, this progression is not inevitable. Diabetes may be delayed or prevented by weight reduction, exercise and conditioning, and metformin therapy (DPP). Furthermore, a minority of people with IGT may return to normal glucose tolerance or maintain IGT for no clear reason. However, many progress to frank diabetes and its complications. In type 2 diabetes, as in type 1 diabetes, the complications of retinopathy, nephropathy, and neuropathy may appear as a function of the duration and extent of hyperglycemia. Serious complications include visual difficulties, blindness, renal insufficiency or end-stage renal disease, and amputation. In addition, people with type 2 diabetes are often seriously disabled from coronary heart disease and die prematurely, most often from a cardiovascular cause.

The good news is that recent studies have provided compelling evidence that an aggressive multifactorial approach to the prevention or delay of the microvascular and macrovascular complications of type 2 diabetes will pay great dividends. This approach to therapy is fully discussed in later chapters.

Key Points: Pathophysiology and Natural History of Type 2 Diabetes

Pathophysiology

- ↝ Type 2 diabetes results from insulin deficiency and insulin resistance.
- ↝ It is not clear which is the primary defect.
- ↝ First-phase insulin secretion is diminished at the stage of IGT, resulting in hyperglycemia and subsequent hyperinsulinemia.
- ↝ At the stage of fasting hyperglycemia, the pancreas has lost 60–75% of its ability to secrete insulin.
- ↝ Hepatic glucose output (HGO) increases in direct proportion to the fasting plasma glucose.
- ↝ Increased fasting plasma glucose is caused by increased HGO.
- ↝ Insulin resistance is accentuated by prolonged hyperglycemia ("glucose toxicity") and is partially reversed by intensive therapy
- ↝ Therapy for type 2 diabetes should be tailored to the underlying defects: decreased insulin secretion (use insulin providers), increased insulin resistance (use insulin sensitizers), and increased hepatic glucose output (use HGO suppression)
- ↝ Combination therapy, directed at multiple sites, is often indicated.

Natural history

- Type 2 diabetes has a strong genetic component. The disorder is polygenic; many candidate genes are under study.
- Major environmental influences are overweight, obesity, and sedentary lifestyle.
- Risk of progression from IGT to frank diabetes can be reduced substantially by an intensive diet and exercise program.

Key Points (*Continued*)

- Before the diagnosis of diabetes, many type 2 diabetics have a constellation of cardiovascular risk factors, termed syndrome X, insulin resistance syndrome, or metabolic syndrome.
- Centripetal obesity, insulin resistance, dyslipidemia, IGT, hypertension, microalbuminuria, and clotting abnormalities occur in various combinations in this syndrome.
- Macrovascular complications relate to many components of this syndrome.
- Microvascular complications relate to prolonged hyperglycemia and hypertension.

Complications

An understanding of the pathogenesis and natural history of the microvascular and macrovascular complication of type 2 diabetes is critical to define and assess sensible and effective therapeutic approaches. This section briefly considers these issues as they concern the major microvascular complications of retinopathy, nephropathy, and neuropathy as well as the major macrovascular complications of myocardial infarctions, strokes, and cardiovascular deaths. Major risk factors and predictors of accelerated rates of cardiovascular disease in type 2 diabetes are discussed. The result is intended to be a framework to allow interpretation of evidence from prospective clinical trials that will support a multifactorial approach to the prevention of progression of micro- and macrovascular disease in people with type 2 diabetes mellitus.

Retinopathy

Many aspects of diabetic retinopathy are common to people with type 1 and type 2 diabetes. The discussion of type 1 diabetes concentrated on the findings from the DCCT, which demonstrated that intensive glucose control can significantly reduce the rate of progression of diabetic retinopathy. This section includes a more thorough discussion of the stages of retinopathy, principal clinical findings, natural history, and guidelines for care for people with type 2 diabetes. Because this disease is substantially more common than type 1 diabetes, its proper management has a significantly greater impact on overall diabetic care. The many stages in the progression of diabetic retinopathy[4,7] are given in Table 2.

It is apparent that precise recognition of these various stages requires specialized training, as does the decision about laser photocoagulation or other forms of therapy. A review of this specialized area is beyond the scope of this book. As previously covered in the discussion of guidelines

Table 2. Stages of Diabetic Retinopathy	
Stage	**Principal Clinical Findings**
Early stages	Retinal vascular microaneurysms and blot hemorrhages
Mild NPDR	Increased retinal vascular permeability
	Cotton wool spots
Middle stages	Venous caliber changes or beading
Moderate NPDR	IRMA
Severe NPDR	Retinal capillary loss
Very severe NPDR	Retinal ischemia
	Extensive intraretinal hemorrhages and microaneurysms
Advanced stages	NVD
PDR	NVE
	Neovascularization of the iris
	Neovascular glaucoma
	Preretinal and vitreous hemorrhage
	Fibrovascular proliferation
	Retinal traction, retinal tears, retinal detachment

NPDR = Non proliferative diabetic retinopathy, PDR = Proliferative diabetic retinopathy, IRMA = Intra-retinal microvascular abnormality, NVD = Neovascularization near the optic disc, NVE = Neovascularization ≥1 disc diameter from the optic disc.

for care,[7] referral for regular dilated eye examinations by an eye specialist is a standard of good primary care. Several aspects of retinopathy in type 2 diabetes differ from findings in type 1 diabetic patients. First, because of the usual delay in the diagnosis of type 2 diabetes, retinopathy is often found at the time of diagnosis.[26,29,30] In the UKPDS, about 37% of freshly diagnosed type 2 diabetics already had retinopathy by retinal photography.[57] Projections have been made from natural history curves, which suggest that hyperglycemia, the hallmark of diabetes, starts at least 4–7 years before the diagnosis of type 2 diabetes is usually made.[26] The diagnostic level of fasting plasma glucose was changed from ≥ 140 mg/dl to ≥ 126 mg/dl because the lower level was shown in a number of studies to be predictive of the eventual development of diabetic retinopathy.[58] On the other hand, retinopathy in type 2 diabetes may not be apparent even in patients with disease of long duration. Data from the Wisconsin Epidemiologic Study of Diabetic Retinopathy (WESDR) showed that only about 60% of diabetic adults (over age 30) who were not receiving insulin had evidence of retinopathy after 25 years of diabetes, and a very small percentage (10% less) had proliferative retinopathy.[29,30] In older diabetics who were treated with insulin because of more severe diabetes, over 80% had retinopathy after 15 years, and about 10% had proliferative retinopathy. Over 20% had retinopathy at the time of diagnosis of type 2 diabetes. Close to 100% of type 1 diabetics have retinopathy after about 15 years, and approximately 25% develop proliferative retinopathy. Because type 2 diabetes is much more prevalent than type 1 diabetes, diabetes is the leading cause of new cases of legal blindness in Americans between the ages of 20 and 74 years.

The impact of this complication is enormous. There are an estimated 700,000 people in the U.S with PDR and 130,000 with high-risk PDR. Vision is threatened, and visual loss may be prevented. Many other treatable conditions that are a threat to vision are shown in Table 3.[4]

It is estimated that 500,000 diabetics have macular edema and that 300,000 have clinically significant macular edema in the U.S. In 1994 it was estimated that appropriate treatment for the retinal complications of type 2 diabetes would generate annual savings of close to $250 million/year and 53,986 person-years of sight.

An understanding of the chances of progression from NPDR to PDR puts in perspective the need for frequent dilated eye examinations in people with diabetes. Thus, as is shown in Table 4, mild NPDR has a 16% chance of progression to high-risk PDR within 5 years, whereas very severe NPDR has a 45% chance of progression in 1 year and a 71% chance of progression in 5 years.[4] Intervention in such patients by retinal specialists is critical to preserve vision.

Table 3. Threats to Vision from Diabetic Retinopathy and Common Initial Treatment

Complication Threatening Vision	Common Initial Treatment
CSME	Focal or grid laser photocoagulation surgery
High-risk PDR	PRP
Vitreous hemorrhage	Careful observation or vitrectomy
Traction and/or retinal detachment	Vitrectomy
Traction distorting macula	Vitrectomy
Neovascular glaucoma	PRP and/or cryotherapy and Intraocular pressure management

PRP = scatter (panretinal) photocoagulation surgery, CSME = clinically significant macular edema, PDR = proliferative diabetic retinopathy.

Table 4. Progression to PDR by NPDR Level

Retinopathy level	Chance of High-risk PDR in 1 Year (%)	Chance of High-risk PDR in 5 Years (%)
Mild NPDR	1	16
Moderate NPDR	3–8	27–39
Severe NPDR	15	56
Very severe NPDR	45	71
PDR with less than high-risk characteristics	22–46	64–75

PDR = proliferative diabetic retinopathy, NPDR = nonproliferative diabetic retinopathy.

Key Points: Retinopathy

↪ Early, middle, and late stages of diabetic retinopathy may occur with increasing duration and poor glycemic control in type 2 diabetes

↪ Stages include mild nonproliferative diabetic retinopathy (NPDR), moderate-to-severe NPDR, and proliferative diabetic retinopathy (PDR)

↪ Yearly examination by an eye specialist is an important standard of care

↪ Retinopathy is found in 20–37% of type 2 diabetics at the time of diagnosis, suggesting that diabetes had been present for 4–7 years before it was diagnosed.

↪ The major rationale behind the choice of FPG ≥ 126 mg/dl for the diagnosis of diabetes is that this level is the cut-off point for predicting the future development of retinopathy

↪ Insulin-treated adult diabetics develop retinopathy that is qualitatively similar to retinopathy in type 1 diabetes. Patients treated with diet are at a lower risk for the development of retinopathy

↪ Appropriate treatment for diabetic retinal complications would save $250 million yearly (1994 data)

↪ A person with mild NPDR has a 16% chance of progressing to PDR in 5 years, whereas a person with very severe NPDR has a 45% chance of progressing in 1 year and a 71% chance of progressing in 5 years.

Nephropathy

The incidence of end-stage renal disease (ESRD) in the U.S. is increasing, and diabetes has become the most common single cause.[6] Diabetic nephropathy accounts for at least one-third of all cases of ESRD, and over 50% of diabetic patients starting on dialysis have type 2 diabetes. Thus, although renal failure is commonly cited as an end stage of diabetic nephropathy in type 1 diabetes, type 2 diabetes is the major overall contributor to ESRD because of its markedly increased prevalence. Furthermore, the incidence of type 2 diabetes is increasing at an alarming rate, and this also contributes to its increased contribution to ESRD among diabetic patients.[5]

The earliest indicator of renal damage in diabetes is the presence of microalbuminuria (≥30mg albumin/24 hr in the urine or a urinary albumin/creatinine ratio ≥30 μg/mg). Microalbuminuria may even precede the diagnosis of type 2 diabetes,[35] and may be seen in the metabolic syndrome as well as in people with impaired glucose tolerance. In contrast to type 1 diabetes, microalbuminuria in type 2 diabetes is a strong predictor of cardiovascular death[15,20,52] and of coronary heart disease[22] but a weaker predictor of renal failure. Microalbuminuria predicts the development of an atherogenic lipoprotein profile in type 2 diabetes.[37,38] The prevalence of microalbuminuria in white type 2 diabetics ranges from 8% to 36%, and in nonwhite diabetics from 26% to 42%. Hypertension and poor glycemic control are major contributing factors, and it is also clear that genetic influences are involved in the development of microalbuminuria. In type 2 diabetes (in contrast to type 1), hypertension is not necessarily associated with microalbuminuria and predicts proteinuria in only a few populations (e.g., the Pima Indians).[36]

The renal lesions in type 2 diabetes are often heterogeneous. In biopsy studies of type 2 diabetic kidneys, 23–31% of biopsies show histologic changes of a nondiabetic nature, and mixed lesions of typical diabetic glomerulosclerosis with nondiabetic glomerular damage (e.g., mesangio-proliferative glomerulonephritis) also may be seen.[21,41] The clinical course of renal disease in type 2 diabetes is not as clearly defined as in type 1 diabetes, in which progressive and typical diabetic glomerulosclerosis is almost always the predominant lesion. It is estimated that about one-third of cases of ESRD in type 2 diabetes are primarily of nondiabetic origin. If a diabetic patient has evidence of nephropathy, the presence of retinopathy suggests that diabetic glomerulopathy is the most likely cause. In a diabetic patient with nephropathy, if retinopathy is absent after careful examination by an eye specialist, a nondiabetic cause of renal damage must be suspected. Renal biopsy is usually needed to make the differentiation.

Without intervention, about 20–40% of type 2 diabetic patients with microalbuminuria progress to macroalbuminuria (>300 mg albumin/day) or overt nephropathy; yet, by 20 years later, only about 20% of these patients have progressed to ESRD.[5] Changes in glomerular filtration rates are often variable. One reason for the difference in the natural history of nephropathy in type 1 and type 2 diabetes may be the increased cardiovascular risk in type 2 diabetes. Thus, death from coronary artery disease obviously prevents the patient from progressing to ESRD.

Key Points: Nephropathy

⟳ Diabetes is the most frequent cause of ESRD, and the incidence is increasing.

⟳ Over 50% of new patients starting dialysis have type 2 diabetes.

⟳ Microalbuminuria (≥30 mg albumin/24 hour urine) is the earliest indicator of renal damage in type 2 diabetes.

⟳ Microalbuminuria may precede type 2 diabetes and is frequently a component of the metabolic syndrome.

Key Points (*Continued*)

⟿ Microalbuminuria is a strong predictor of cardiovascular death in type 2 diabetes and a weak predictor of renal failure.

⟿ Prevalence of microalbuminuria range from 8% to 36% in white type 2 diabetics and is higher (26–42%) in nonwhite diabetics.

⟿ Hypertension is not necessarily associated with microalbuminuria in type 2 diabetes.

⟿ In contrast to type 1 diabetes, 23–31% of renal biopsies in people with type 2 diabetes show nondiabetic lesions.

⟿ The presence of retinopathy suggests that nephropathy in type 2 diabetes is of diabetic origin.

⟿ If retinopathy is absent, renal biopsy is needed for accurate diagnosis of the renal lesion.

⟿ Without intervention, about 20–40% of type 2 diabetics with microalbuminuria will progress to macroalbuminuria and 20% to ESRD.

Neuropathy

Peripheral sensory polyneuropathy is present in 5–10% of people at the time of diagnosis of type 2 diabetes. In prospective studies with standard management, 40–50% have evidence of peripheral sensory neuropathy after 10 years of type 2 diabetes.[40] The diagnosis is usually made by a careful history and physical examination. The symptoms of peripheral sensory polyneuropathy in diabetes are listed in Table 5.[53] Significant physical findings may suggest the presence of peripheral sensory polyneuropathy (Table 6).[53] Finally, the diagnosis may be confirmed by sensory testing with simple, user-friendly instruments (Table 7).[53]

Table 5. Symptoms of Peripheral Sensory Polyneuropathy

Sensory symptoms
Numbness or dead feeling in the feet
"Pins and needles" (paresthesia) in the feet
Pain in the legs: stabbing, shooting, burning, or deep aching
Unusual sensations: "tightly wrapped" feeling around the foot, "cotton wool" feeling under the toes
Contact hypersensitivity
Inability to identify objects in the hands
Unsteadiness of gait
Motor symptoms
Difficulty walking or climbing stairs
Difficulty lifting objects
Difficulty handling small objects

Table 6. Signs of Peripheral Sensory Polyneuropathy
Inspection
Normal feet may be present
Dry skin, distended veins, edema (autonomic features)
Deformities: neuropathic clawing, hallux valgus, Charcot joint
Muscle atrophy
Callus formation
Foot ulceration
Gait disturbance/ataxia
Examination
Warm, dry feet
Bounding foot pulses
Loss , or reduction, of knee and ankle tendon reflexes
Loss of ankle dorsiflexion

The 10-gram monofilament is used to assess pressure sensation and has been shown to be a good test for predicting ulceration. Insensitivity is defined as no sensation after a force sufficient to cause the filament to buckle. Generally, testing is done on at least one of four plantar sites on the forefoot, including the great toe and the first, third, and fifth metatarsal heads. Decreased to absent vibration sensation, as assessed by a tuning fork over the great toe or malleoli, is also a predictor of ulceration.

Numerous cross-sectional studies have been done in attempts to define risk factors for peripheral sensory polyneuropathy. Longitudinal studies, although less numerous, are preferable for multivariate analysis. In the Seattle Prospective Foot Study, hyperglycemia was a predictor of monofilament insensitivity.[2,8] There was a 15% increase in risk for each 1% increase in HbA1c. In a prospective study of type 2 diabetics in Finland, glycemia was a predictor of peripheral sensory polyneuropathy.[40] Evidence from the UKPDS and the Kumomoto Study[39] that intensive glycemic management delays progression of sensory neuropathy in type 2 diabetes lends strong support to the concept that hyperglycemia is the predominant risk factor for peripheral sensory polyneuropathy. Other

Table 7. Sensory Modality Testing	
Sensory Modality	Instrument Used for Testing
Pressure sensation	10-gm monofilament
Pain sensation	Disposable neuro-tips
Vibration sensation	128-Hz tuning fork
Cold sensation	Cold tuning fork
Light touch	Wisp of cotton

risk markers include age, height, ethnicity (American Indians), alcohol abuse, and increased urinary albumin excretion.[1]

Foot Ulceration

Peripheral sensory neuropathy and peripheral vascular disease are predictors of foot ulceration in people with diabetes.[1] A history of previous ulceration markedly increases the risk of subsequent foot ulceration. Elevated plantar foot pressures are present in patients who develop ulceration and are usually associated with plantar callus. Callus, in turn, is a risk factor for foot ulceration. Minor trauma had occurred in 77% of all patients with foot ulcers in one study, making it an important risk marker. Thus, a number of risk factors or markers increase the probability of foot ulceration. They can be determined by simple examination. Identification of patients at high risk for foot ulceration should lead to preventive measures, which have been shown to be effective in prevention of the serious complication of amputation.

Autonomic Neuropathy

The other major category of neuropathy in diabetes is autonomic neuropathy.[63] It is associated with a reduced quality of life as well as poor prognosis. The clinical manifestations of diabetic autonomic neuropathy may involve a variety of systems:[63]

- **Cardiovascular:** resting tachycardia, orthostatic hypotension, sudden death.
- **Respiratory:** sleep apnea, reduced ventilatory drive.
- **Gastrointestinal:** esophageal dysfunction, gastroparesis, diabetic diarrhea, constipation,
- **Genitourinary:** neurogenic gallbladder, erectile dysfunction, retrograde ejaculation.
- **Sudomotor:** hypohidrosis, gustatory sweating.
- **Vasomotor:** Vasodilatation, edema.
- **Neuroendocrine:** defective counter-regulation to hypoglycemia, hypoglycemia unawareness.

Diabetic autonomic neuropathy is particularly associated with long-term diabetes and poor metabolic control. Occasionally however, it is seen in newly diagnosed type 1 diabetic patients. Prevalence varies among studies, and it may be slightly less common in type 2 than in type 1 diabetic patients. In one study, evidence of autonomic neuropathy was present in 21% of type 1 patients and 6% of type 2 diabetic individuals. Other studies have found approximately equal prevalence rates in the two types of diabetes, ranging from 8% to 22%. In any case, although a relatively rare complication, it has devastating consequences.

Key Points: Neuropathy

⊷ Peripheral sensory polyneuropathy is present in 5–10% of people with diabetes at the time of diagnosis and in 40–50% after 10 years of standard management.

⊷ Symptoms and signs of peripheral sensory polyneuropathy are characteristic (Tables 5 and 6).

⊷ Simple testing with 1.0-gram monofilament, tuning fork, and/or cotton tips confirms the diagnosis.

⊷ Hyperglycemia is the major risk factor for peripheral sensory polyneuropathy.

⊷ For each 1% increase of HbA1c, there is a 15% increase in the risk for monofilament insensitivity of the feet.

⊷ Other risk markers for peripheral sensory neuropathy are age, height, alcohol abuse, ethnicity (American Indians), and microalbuminuria.

⊷ Peripheral sensory neuropathy and peripheral vascular disease are risk markers for foot ulceration.

⊷ A history of a previous ulcer markedly increases the risk for subsequent foot ulceration.

⊷ Callus often precedes ulceration and usually is associated with elevated plantar foot pressures.

⊷ Minor trauma precedes foot ulceration in 77% of cases.

⊷ Autonomic neuropathy affecting the cardiovascular, gastrointestinal, genitourinary, and/or neuroendocrine systems often leads to devastating consequences in people with diabetes.

⊷ Autonomic neuropathy is particularly associated with long-term diabetes and poor metabolic control.

⊷ Evidence of autonomic neuropathy is found in approximately 21% of type 1 and 6% of type 2 diabetics.

Macrovascular Complications

Cardiovascular Death

Accelerated complications of atherosclerotic cardiovascular disease occur in the majority of patients with type 2 diabetes.[12,55,56] Epidemiologic studies indicate that the risk of cardiovascular mortality is 2–3 times higher in men with type 2 diabetes[55] and 3–5 times higher in women with type 2 diabetes[32] than in people without diabetes. This increased risk may be present before diabetes[25] and is multiplied significantly by the presence of hypertension, microalbuminuria, dyslipidemia, cigarette smoking, and components of the metabolic syndrome.[28,56] The metabolic syndrome may include a prothrombotic tendency, which appears to be related to increased plasma fibrinogen levels; increased activity of plasminogen activator inhibitor (PAI-1), which is an inhibitor of the fibrinolytic system; and increased platelet adhesiveness, aggregation, and thromboxane production.[11,12] The net result has been a markedly decreased life expectancy of 5–10 years in people with type 2 diabetes due to cardiovascular events.

Although there has been an overall steady decrease in cardiovascular mortality in the U.S. over the past few decades, no similar decrease has been seen in type 2 diabetics. A recent study analyzed mortality in men and women in the first National Health and Nutrition Examination Survey (NHANES I).[23] Two cohorts of diabetic patients in the study were followed for 8.7 or 9.1 years in two separate decades: early 1980s and early 1990s. Cardiovascular mortality decreased significantly among nondiabetic men and women when the two cohorts were compared. Decrease was minimal in diabetic men, and mortality from heart disease actually rose by 10–22% in diabetic women in the two decades studied. The authors concluded that one reason for the difference between nondiabetics and diabetics may have been that preventive measures were used more extensively or provided more benefit to people without type 2 diabetes than to those with the disease. Evidence indicates that optimal control of cardiovascular risk factors is achieved only in a minority of patients, even in urban academic medical centers.

Haffner et al. compared the cardiovascular mortality rates of nondiabetics who had suffered a myocardial infarction and type 2 diabetics who had no history of myocardial infarction.[24] This study demonstrated that the prognosis for cardiovascular death is the same for a type 2 diabetic who has had no history of a heart attack as it is for an age- and gender-matched nondiabetic who has already had a myocardial infarction. Recognition of this fact, along with other epidemiologic evidence, helped persuade the National Cholesterol Education Program group to elevate type 2 diabetes to the level of a cardiovascular risk equivalent: equal to elevated plasma cholesterol, cigarette smoking, and strong family history of cardiovascular disease.[17] Thus, aggressive cardiovascular risk reduction strategies are recommended for all people with type 2 diabetes.

Predictors of Cardiovascular Mortality in Type 2 Diabetes

Insight into which of the many cardiovascular risk markers to emphasize is provided by long-term epidemiologic observations of people with type 2 diabetes. In one unique study, a 15-year follow-up of type 2 diabetics was compared with a nondiabetic control group.[37] As was true in older studies, both men and women with type 2 diabetes had markedly increased odds ratios for cardiovascular mortality. Hyperglycemia was a predictor of cardiovascular mortality, as shown in the UKPDS and many other studies. A major finding was that lipoprotein abnormalities, which are characteristic of type 2 diabetes, were strong predictors of cardiovascular events. These abnormalities included low plasma HDL-cholesterol and increased triglyceride concentration, increased apolipoprotein B level, and low LDL cholesterol-to-apolipoprotein B ratio. The last finding is indicative of the fact that small, dense LDL particles rather than high LDL cholesterol concentrations are predictors of cardiovascular events in type 2 diabetes.

Elevated blood pressure is more common in people with type 2 diabetes than in a control population. The UKPDS, conclusively demonstrated that systolic blood pressure had a significant correlation with both microvascular and macrovascular complications of diabetes.[3] No threshold of systolic blood pressure was observed for the increased risk. Other studies have shown a relationship between elevated blood pressure and cardiovascular death in people with type 2 diabetes.[54,55] Hypertension is a risk factor for albuminuria and diabetic nephropathy, and both conditions are associated with high cardiovascular mortality as well as end-stage renal disease.

Other cardiovascular risk factors are important in type 2 diabetes. In the Nurses' Health Study, cigarette smoking was associated in a dose-response fashion with increased mortality among women with type 2 diabetes.[48] Furthermore smoking cessation appeared to decrease this risk substantially. Microalbuminuria is a predictor of cardiovascular events and death in type 2 diabetes. Fibrinogen is established as a cardiovascular risk factor in nondiabetic and diabetic individuals.[9,11,12] Recently, another marker of inflammation, highly sensitive C-reactive protein, has been implicated as a predictor of cardiovascular events.[49,50] Elevation of these acute-phase reactants in analyzed plasma from diabetics has fostered new interest in the possibility that a vascular inflammatory process may underlie accelerated atherosclerosis in people with diabetes.[51]

Other factors that may be involved in the pathogenesis of atherosclerosis in diabetes have been described. Many alterations in platelet function are thought to contribute to a prothrombotic state. Fibrinolysis is often defective in type 2 diabetes, and this prothrombotic tendency has been attributed, at least in part, to elevated plasma PAI-1 levels.[11,12] Homocysteine levels may be elevated in the plasma of people with the metabolic syndrome[34] and in type 2 diabetes[16,18] particularly in the presence of renal damage.[10] Plasma homocysteine is a predictor of accelerated vascular disease.

Thus, many factors may contribute to the rapid rate of progression of atherosclerosis and its complications in type 2 diabetes. Another section focuses on the intervention trials that give encouraging information about how to structure an intensive management strategy in type 2 diabetes that will achieve the best possible outcomes.

References

1. Adler A: Risk factors for diabetic neuropathy and foot ulceration. Curr Diabetes Rep I:202–207, 2001.
2. Adler AI, Boyko EJ, Ahroni JH, et al: Risk factors for diabetic peripheral sensory neuropathy. Diabetes Care 20:1162–1167, 1997.
3. Adler AI, Stratton IM, Neil AW, et al: Association of systolic blood pressure with macrovascular and microvascular complications of type 2 diabetes (UKPDS 36): prospective observational study. BMJ 321:412–419, 2000.
4. Aiello LP, Gardner TW, King GL, et al: Diabetic retinopathy. Diabetes Care 21:143–156, 1998.
5. Alzaid AA: Microalbuminuria in patients with NIDDM: An overview. Diabetes Care 19:79–89, 1996.
6. American Diabetes Association: Diabetic nephropathy. Diabetes Care 25:S85–S89, 2002.
7. American Diabetes Association: Diabetic retinopathy. Diabetes Care 25:S90–S93, 2002.
8. Boyko E, Ahroni J, Stensel V, et al: A prospective study of risk factors for diabetic foot ulcer. The Seattle Diabetic Foot Study. Diabetes Care 22:1036–1042, 1999.
9. Ceriello A: Fibrinogen and diabetes mellitus: Is it time for intervention trial? Diabetologia 40:731–734, 1997.
10. Colwell JA: Elevated plasma homocysteine and diabetic vascular disease [editorial]. Diabetes Care 20:1805–1806, 1997.
11. Colwell JA: Treatment for the procoagulant state in type 2 diabetes. Endocrinol Metab Clin North Am 30:1011–1030, 2001.
12. Colwell JA, Jokl R: Vascular thrombosis in diabetes. In Porte D, Sherwin R, Rifkin H. (eds): Diabetes Mellitus: Theory and Practice, 5th ed. Norwalk, CT: Appleton Lange, 1996, pp 207–216.
13. DeFronzo RA: Pathogenesis of type 2 (non-insulin-dependent) diabetes mellitus: a balanced overview. Diabetologia 35:389–397, 1992.
14. Diabetes Prevention Program Research Group: Reduction in the incidence of type 2 diabetes with lifestyle intervention or metformin. N Engl J Med 346:393–403, 2002.
15. Dinneen SF, Gerstein HC: The association of microalbuminuria and mortality in non-insulin-dependent diabetes mellitus. A systematic overview of the literature. Arch Intern Med 157:1413–1418, 1997.
16. Drzewoski J, Czupryniak L, Chwatko G, et al: Hyperhomocysteinemia in poorly controlled Type 2 diabetes patients. Diabetes Nutr Metab 13:319–324, 2000.
17. Executive Summary of the Third Report of the National Cholesterol Education Program (NCEP) Expert Panel on Detection, Evaluation, and Treatment of High Blood Cholesterol in Adults (Adult Treatment Panel III). JAMA 285:2486–2497, 2001.
18. Fonseca VA, Reynolds T, Fink LM: Hyperhomocysteinemia and microalbuminuria in diabetes. Diabetes Care 21:1028, 1998.
19. Ford ES, Giles WH, Dietz WH, et al: Prevalence of the metabolic syndrome among US adults: Findings from the third national health and nutrition examination survey. JAMA 287:356–359, 2002.
20. Gall MA, Borch-Johnsen K, Hougaard P, et al: Albuminuria and poor glycemic control predict mortality in NIDDM. Diabetes 44:1303–1309, 1995.

21. Gambara V, Mecca G, Remuzzi G, et al: Heterogeneous nature of renal lesions in type II diabetes. J Am Soc Nephrol 3:1458–1466, 1993.
22. Gerstein HC, Mann JFE, Yi Q, et al: Albuminuria and risk of cardiovascular events, death, and heart failure in diabetic and nondiabetic individuals. JAMA 286:421–426, 2001.
23. Gu K, Cowie CC, Harris MI: Diabetes and decline in heart disease mortality in US adults. JAMA 281:1291–1297, 1999.
24. Haffner SM, Lehto S, Ronnemaa T, et al: Mortality from coronary heart disease in subjects with type 2 diabetes and in nondiabetic subjects with and without prior myocardial infarction. N Engl J Med 339:229–234, 1998.
25. Haffner SM, Stern MP, Hazuda HP, et al: Cardiovascular risk factors in confirmed prediabetic individuals. Does the clock for coronary heart disease start ticking before the onset of clinical diabetes? JAMA 263:2893–2898, 1990.
26. Harris MI, Klein R, Welborn TA, et al: Onset of NIDDM occurs at least 4–7 yr before clinical diagnosis. Diabetes 15:815–819, 1992.
27. Helmrich SP, Ragland DR, Leung RW, et al: Physical activity and reduced occurrence of non-insulin-dependent diabetes mellitus. N Engl J Med 325:147–152, 1991.
28. Isomaa B, Almbfen P, Tuomi T, et al: Cardiovascular morbidity and mortality associated with the metabolic syndrome. Diabetes Care 24:683–689, 2001.
29. Klein R: Hyperglycemia and microvascular and macrovascular disease in diabetes. Diabetes Care 18:258–268, 1995.
30. Klein R, Klein BEK, Moss SE, et al: The Wisconsin Epidemiologic Study of Diabetic Retinopathy: III. Prevalence and risk of diabetic retinopathy when age at diagnosis is 30 or more years. Arch Ophthalmol 102:527–532, 1984.
31. Lillioja S, Mott DM,, Spraul M, et al: Insulin resistance and insulin secretory dysfunction as precursors of non-insulin-dependent diabetes mellitus. Prospective Studies of Pima Indians. N Engl J Med 329:1988–1992, 1993.
32. Manson JE, Colditz GA, Stampfer MJ, et al: A prospective study of maturity-onset diabetes mellitus and risk of coronary heart disease and stroke in women. Arch Intern Med 151:1141–1147, 1991.
33. Mattock MB, Barnes DJ, Viberti GC, et al: Microalbuminuria and coronary heart disease in NIDDM. An Incidence study. Diabetes 47:1786–1792, 1998.
34. Meigs, JB, Jacques PF, Selhub, J, et al: Fasting plasma homocysteine levels in the insulin resistance syndrome. Diabetes Care 24:1403–1410, 2001.
35. Mykkänen L, Haffner SM, Juusisto J, et al: Microalbuminuria precedes the development of NIDDM. Diabetes 43:552–557, 1994.
36. Nelson RG, Knowler WC, Pettitt DJ, et al: Diabetic kidney disease in the Pima Indians. Diabetes Care 16 (Suppl 1):335–341, 1993.
37. Niskanen L, Turpeinen A, Penttila I, et al: Hyperglycemia and compositional lipoprotein abnormalities as predictors of cardiovascular mortality in type 2 diabetes: A 15-year follow-up from the time of diagnosis. Diabetes Care 21:1861–1869, 1998.
38. Niskanen L, Uusitupa M, Sarlund H, et al: Microalbuminuria predicts the development of serum lipoprotein abnormalities favouring atherogenesis in newly diagnosed type 2 (non-insulin-dependent) diabetic patients. Diabetologia 33:237–243, 1990.
39. Ohkubo Y, Kishikawa H, Araki E, et al: Intensive insulin therapy prevents the progression of diabetic microvascular complications in Japanese patients with non-insulin-dependent diabetes mellitus: a randomized prospective 6-year study. Diabetes Res Clin Pract 28:103–117, 1995.
40. Partanen J, Niskanen L, Lehtinen J, et al: Natural history of peripheral neuropathy in

patients with non-insulin-dependent diabetes mellitus. N Engl J Med 333:89–94, 1995.

41. Parving HH: Renoprotection in diabetes: genetic and non-genetic risk factors and treatment. Diabetologia 41:745–759, 1998.

42. Pimenta W, Korytkowski M, Mitrakou A, et al: Pancreatic beta-cell dysfunction as the primary genetic lesion in NIDDM. Evidence from studies in normal glucose-tolerant individuals with a first-degree NIDDM Relative. JAMA 273:1855–1861, 1995.

43. Polonsky KS, Sturis J, Bell, GI: Non-insulin-dependent diabetes mellitus: A genetically programmed failure of the beta cell to compensate for insulin resistance. N Engl J Med 334:777–783, 1996.

44. Porte J: Banting Lecture 1990. β-Cells in type II diabetes mellitus. Diabetes 40:166–180, 1991.

45. Pratley RE, Weyer C: The role of impaired early insulin secretion in the pathogenesis of type II diabetes mellitus. Diabetologia 44:929–945, 2001.

46. Reaven GM: Role of insulin resistance in human disease. Diabetes 37:1595–1607, 1988.

47. Rich-Edwards JW, Colditz GA, Stampfer MJ: Birth weight and the risk for type 2 diabetes mellitus in adult women. Ann Intern Med 130:278–284, 1999.

48. Rich-Edwards JW, Manson JE, Hennekens CH, et al: The primary prevention of coronary heart disease in women. N Engl J Med 332:1758–1766, 1995.

49. Ridker PM, Hennekens CH, Buring JE, et al: C-reactive protein and other markers of inflammation in the prediction of cardiovascular disease in women. N Engl J Med 342:836–843, 2000.

50. Ridker PM, Cushman M, Stampfer MJ, et al: Inflammation, aspirin, and the risk of cardiovascular disease in apparently healthy men. N Engl J Med 336:973–979, 1997.

51. Ross R. Atherosclerosis—an inflammatory disease. N Engl J Med 340:115–126, 1999.

52. Schmitz, A, Vaeth M: Microalbuminuria: A major risk factor in non-insulin-dependent diabetes. A 10-year follow-up study of 503 patients. Diabetic Medicine 5:126–134, 1988.

53. Scott LA, Tesfaye S: Measurement of somatic neuropathy for clinical practice and clinical trials. Current Diabetes Reports I:208–215, 2001.

54. Stamler J, Stamler R, Neaton JD. Blood pressure, systolic and diastolic, and cardiovascular risks: US population data. Arch Intern Med 153:598–615, 1993.

55. Stamler J, Vaccaro O, Neaton JD, et al: Diabetes, other risk factors, and 12-yr cardiovascular mortality for men screened in the multiple risk factor intervention trial. Diabetes Care 16:434–444, 1993.

56. Stern M: Perspectives in diabetes: Diabetes and cardiovascular disease. The "common soil" hypothesis. Diabetes 44:369–374, 1995.

57. Stratton IM, Kohner EM, Aldington SJ, et al: UKPDS 50: Risk factors for incidence and progression of retinopathy in type II diabetes over 6 years from diagnosis. Diabetologia 44:156–163, 2001.

58. The Expert Committee on the Diagnosis and Classification of Diabetes Mellitus: Report of the expert committee on the diagnosis and classification of diabetes mellitus. Diabetes Care 20:1183–1197,1997.

59. Tuomilehto J, Lindstrom J, Eriksson JG, et l: Prevention of type 2 diabetes mellitus by changes in lifestyle among subjects with impaired glucose tolerance. N Engl J Med 344:1343–1350, 2001.

60. Yalow RS, Berson SA: Immunoassay of endogenous plasma insulin in man. J Clin Invest 39:1157–1175, 1960.

61. Yki-Järvinen H: Pathogenesis of non-insulin-dependent diabetes mellitus. Lancet 343:91–95, 1994.

62. Yki-Järvinen H: Role of insulin resistance in the pathogenesis of NIDDM. Diabetologia 38:1378–1388, 1995.

63. Ziegler D: Diagnosis and treatment of diabetic autonomic neuropathy. Curr Diabetes Rep I:216–227, 2001.

Delaying the Onset of Type 2 Diabetes

chapter
9

As previously discussed, many people with type 2 diabetes have impaired glucose tolerance (IGT) before the onset of fasting hyperglycemia. According to the Third National Health and Nutrition Examination Survey (NHANES III), which was carried out in 1988–1994, 15.6% of people between the ages of 40 and 74 years had IGT by oral glucose tolerance testing. The prevalence of IGT increased with age and was more common in Mexican-Americans (20.2%) than in blacks (14.0%) or whites (15.3%).[2] It is likely that these figures would be higher in a more current survey in view of the increasing incidence of obesity in the U.S.[3]

IGT is a predictor of increased cardiovascular morbidity and mortality. It is frequently seen in the metabolic syndrome and may coexist with hypertension, dyslipidemia, microalbuminuria, and a hypercoagulable state. Longitudinal studies have shown that people with IGT are 50% more likely to die during long-term follow-up than people with normal glucose tolerance. Cardiovascular death is the leading cause. People with IGT may revert to normal glucose tolerance, continue with IGT, or progress to diabetes. Prospective studies have shown that 3.8–8.7% of people with IGT progress to diabetes each year. The main risk factors for progression are obesity and physical inactivity.

Two large-scale prospective trials, one in Finland[4] and one in the United States,[1] have shown a 58% reduction in the risk of progressing from IGT to fasting hyperglycemia (diabetes) if intensive diet and exercise programs are successfully implemented in overweight patients. In the Diabetes Prevention Program in the U.S., the group assigned to intensive lifestyle intervention lost 5–7% of body weight and averaged 30 minutes of moderate-intensity exercise daily. In 3 years, 29% of the control group progressed to diabetes, whereas only 14% of the intensive management group developed diabetes. Improvement in insulin sensitivity is the most likely mechanism. Of note, the average body mass index in this study was in the obesity range ($34kg/m^2$), and that average weight loss was modest. It is not clear without prolonged follow-up whether diabetes is permanently prevented or whether its onset is simply delayed. In either case it is expected that progression to the long-term vascular complications of type 2 diabetes will be delayed in the intensively managed groups.

The progression from IGT to diabetes also may be prevented or delayed by drug therapy. To date, the largest study of the use of an insulin sensitizer (metformin) is the Diabetes Prevention Program (DPP). The group randomly assigned to metformin therapy (850 mg twice daily) had a risk reduction of 31%. Although somewhat less than the 58% observed in the group with intensive lifestyle changes, these results are promising, for they indicate that a pharmacologic approach may successfully prevent or delay the onset of type 2 diabetes.

Other studies will follow. The thiazolidinediones are insulin sensitizers and may prove to be as effective as lifestyle changes or metformin therapy. In the Heart Outcomes Prevention Evaluation (HOPE) Trial, the effect of ramipril, an angiotensin-converting enzyme (ACE) inhibitor, on the development of diabetes in people over age 55 who had vascular disease was studied.[5] With a mean follow-up of 4.5 years, 3.6% in the ramipril group and 5.4% in the placebo group developed diabetes. Relative risk was 0.66 ($p < 0.001$). An effect of ACE inhibitor therapy on insulin resistance is one postulated mechanism. This study has stimulated development of a new large prospective trial, Diabetes Reduction Assessment with Ramipril and Rosiglitazone Medication (DREAM), in people with impaired glucose tolerance to evaluate prospectively whether these drugs prevent or delay the onset of type 2 diabetes. Another large multicenter trial will explore whether a combination of an ACE inhibitor (valsartan) with a meglitinide (nataglinide): to stimulate immediate insulin release will prevent or delay onset of type 2 diabetes in people with IGT. This trial is termed the Nateglinide and Valsartin in Impaired Glucose Tolerance Outcomes Research (NAVIGATOR) Trial.

It is obvious that there is great interest in developing approaches to prevent people from progressing from IGT to diabetes. This work has tremendous public health importance in view of the high prevalence of IGT and its devasting cardiovascular outcomes. Very early diagnosis and treatment of people at high risk for developing diabetes are likely to become a standard of care in future years.

References

1. Diabetes Prevention Program Research Group: Reduction in the incidence of type 2 diabetes with lifestyle intervention or metformin. N Engl J Med 346:393–403, 2002.
2. Harris MI, Flegal KM, Cowie CC, et al: Prevalence of diabetes, impaired fasting glucose, and impaired glucose tolerance in U.S. adults. Diabetes Care 21:518–524, 1998.
3. Mokdad AH, Bowman BA, Ford ES, et al: The continuing epidemics of obesity and diabetes in the United States. JAMA 286:1195–1200, 2001.

4. Tuomilehto J, Lindstrom J, Eriksson JG, et al: Prevention of type 2 diabetes mellitus by changes in lifestyle among subjects with impaired glucose tolerance. N Engl J Med 344:1343–1350, 2001.
5. Yusuf S, Gerstein H, Hoogwerf B, et al: Ramipril and the development of diabetes. JAMA 286:1882–1885, 2001.

Intensive Management of Type 2 Diabetes

chapter 10

Hyperglycemia

Pathophysiology

Type 2 diabetes is characterized by a combination of insulin resistance and diminished insulin secretion. Pathophysiologically, it is quite different from type 1 diabetes, in which severe insulin deficiency or complete lack of insulin production predominates. In addition, type 2 diabetes is a progressive disorder. Insulin resistance may change in either direction. With successful nutrition therapy and an exercise program, insulin resistance may diminish substantially. Successful glycemic regulation decreases insulin resistance in type 2 diabetes. Drugs of the thiazolidine type and (to a lesser degree) metformin act as insulin sensitizers and thereby increase insulin sensitivity.

At the time of diagnosis of type 2 diabetes, beta cell function is diminished, and with increasing duration insulin release by the pancreas gradually diminishes because of depletion of insulin stored in the pancreas (Fig. 1, Chapter 8). Insulin release may be responsive to insulin secretagogues, but the defect is often so profound, particularly in type 2 diabetes of long duration, that insulin therapy is required for intensive glycemic regulation and for partial restoration of insulin sensitivity. During the stages of type 2 diabetes characterized by fasting hyperglycemia, hepatic glucose output is increased. Metformin and insulin therapy are effective in suppressing hepatic glucose output.

Thus, glycemic therapy for people with type 2 diabetes usually proceeds from initial emphasis on diet and exercise to monotherapy, then to combination oral agent therapy, and finally to combination of oral agent(s) and insulin. If the HbA1c target of < 8% is not met after 3 months, the next step should be taken, and this process is continued until the glycemic goal of HbA1c of 7% or less can be met without undue side effects, such as recurrent hypoglycemia.

Figure 2, Chapter 8 gives a perspective on the management of type 2 diabetes. It describes four stages, which can be defined well by prevailing fasting plasma glucose levels. Generally, this progression from phase I to phase IV proceeds as a function of the duration of impaired glucose tolerance and type 2 diabetes. A patient may be first seen at any stage in this sequence. Ideally people at high risk for diabetes would be diagnosed in the stage of impaired glucose tolerance, and vigorously treated to delay or prevent progression. This goal is rarely accomplished at present in the U.S. and will be a major public health problem for diabetic management in the future.[54] At this early stage, insulin resistance is present, first-phase insulin release is diminished, and second-phase release after meals is increased. Hepatic glucose output is normal. Nutritional planning and treatment as well as an exercise conditioning program are critical at this stage and should continue for all stages of type 2 diabetes. However, this approach may not be successful in achieving HbA1c goals, and drug therapy is usually needed. Recent studies support the use of insulin sensitizers (metformin, thiazolidinediones) in the impaired glucose tolerance stage. As the patient progresses to stages II and III, combined oral agent therapy may be effective. Thus, with fasting hyperglycemia between 126 and approximately 200 mg/dl drug treatment often is initiated with an insulin sensitizer. This treatment often results in a HbA1c drop of 1–2%. If the HbA1c goal is not reached, an agent to stimulate insulin secretion (meglitinides or sulfonylureas) is added. An additional fall in HbA1c of 1–2% may occur. It is important to note that the second agent is added to the first agent for this additional effect. This approach addresses the causes of the hyperglycemia at different pathophysiologic sites. If dual oral agent therapy is not successful, addition of an alpha glucosidase inhibitor may give some added benefit (a fall of 0.5–1% in HbA1c). Controlled trials on the use of three or more oral agents in combination, however, are few.

Many physicians choose to add insulin if HbA1c goals are not met by dual therapy with an insulin sensitizer plus an insulin secretagogue. This step can be viewed as phase IV in management. Fasting plasma glucose is consistently greater than 200 mg/dl, and HbA1c is above the 8% action level. At this stage (as shown in Fig. 2, Chapter 8), overall insulin secretion is markedly diminished, and insulin resistance is increased, primarily because of glucose toxicity. Insulin therapy is needed to replace the depleted insulin supply and to diminish glucose toxicity and increase insulin sensitivity by returning plasma glucose levels to nearly normal. The many approaches to the use of oral agents and insulin in type 2 diabetes, are discussed in more detail in future sections.

Evidence for Intensive Glucose Control

Large-scale collaborative trials in the United Kingdom [205] and Japan (Kumamoto Study)[149] have established that intensive glucose management is associated with a diminished rate of development of the microvascular complications of type 2 diabetes: retinopathy, nephropathy, and neuropathy. The risk reductions in retinopathy progression in relation to prevailing HbA1c levels are approximately the same as those seen in intensively managed type 1 patients in the DCCT. Furthermore, retinopathy progression also appeared to follow a curvilinear relation to average HbA1c values in the UKPDS, with no evidence of a glycemic threshold (Fig. 1). Thus, the argument that any diminution in HbA1c

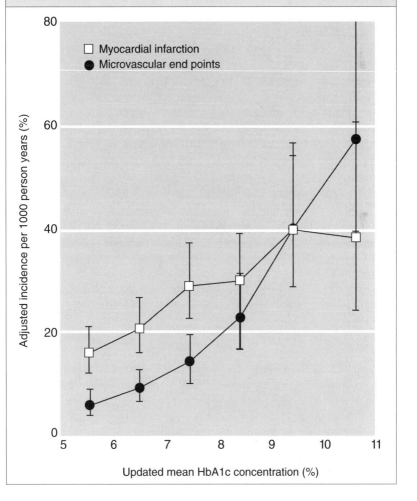

Figure 1. Incidence rates and 95% confidence intervals for microvascular complications and myocardial infarction by category of updated mean HbA1c concentration (%). (From Stratton, IM et al. BMJ 321:405–412, 2000, with permission.)

reduces the risk of progression of diabetic retinopathy applies to type 2 as well as to type 1 diabetes. In these large studies, retinopathy was an objective primary endpoint, and the evidence for intensive glycemic control is therefore strongest for this microvascular complication.

The epidemiologic basis relating hyperglycemia to macrovascular events is solid in the case of established diabetes,[78,112,119,192] and the cardiovascular risk increases with higher prevailing plasma glucose or HbA1c levels.[19,111,120,121,185] Myocardial infarction,[192] all-cause and cardiovascular mortality,[192,211] and stroke have been associated with increasing degrees of hyperglycemia. In the UKPDS, myocardial infarction (MI) risk was doubled in type 2 diabetic men with HbA1c concentrations over 9%, compared with men with levels below 6% (Fig. 1).[192] A 1% decrease in HbA1c appeared to reduce MI risk by 14%. There appears to be no threshold of FPG[47] or of HbA1c levels[192] for cardiovascular events in diabetics.

Many studies have shown that the plasma glucose level after a glucose challenge is a predictor of cardiovascular events or death. Analysis of pooled data from multiple studies of fasting plasma glucose levels in the past gave conflicting results, but more recent meta-analysis indicates that increasing fasting plasma glucose levels in the normal range were associated with increased cardiovascular risk.[47] Compared with a fasting plasma glucose level of 75 mg/dl, a level of 110 mg/dl was associated with a relative cardiovascular event risk of 1.33 (95% CI: 1.06–1.67). More recently, it has become apparent that HbA1c levels are correlated positively with coronary artery disease and carotid artery thickness[217] or stenosis[24] in nondiabetic men and that HbA1c level predicts cardiovascular disease in nondiabetics. In the EPIC-Norfolk study, HbA1c levels had a continuous relationship to cardiovascular risk, even at the normal range of 5–6%.[111]

In contrast, controversy surrounds the effect of intensive glycemic management on the macrovascular complications of diabetes, including myocardial infarction (fatal or nonfatal), sudden death, stroke, peripheral vascular insufficiency, and vascular reconstructive procedures. Five large-scale collaborative trials (Table 1) have explored the effect of intensive vs. standard plasma glucose management in people with type 2 diabetes.

The first study was the University Group Diabetes Program (UGDP),[2] which compared standard insulin therapy with a more intensive insulin management strategy in newly diagnosed type 2 diabetic patients. Despite a mean blood glucose difference of about 50 mg/dl over the course of the 8.75-year follow-up, there was no difference in CVD deaths between the two insulin-treated groups. The United Kingdom Prospective Diabetes Study[205] was also done in newly diagnosed diabetes and compared a standard treatment program with a more intensive strategy. The

Table 1. Studies of Intensive v Standard Glycemic Management in Type 2 Diabetes

Study*	No. of Patients	Mean Age (yr)	Mean Duration of Diabetes (yr)	Study Duration (yr)	FPG or HbA1c Difference	Baseline CVD	CV Event Rate/Yr	Major Results: Cardiovascular Events
UGDP	414	52.7	0	8.75	50 mg/dl	18%	1.4%[†]	No difference in deaths from CVD. (insulin standard vs. insulin intensive)
UKPDS	4209	54	0	10	0.9%	16%	2.0%[‡]	Trend for reduction in MI (p = .052) for policy of intensive treatment. No difference in pooled CV events
Kumamoto	110	49.3	8.4	6	2.3%	0%	0.9%[‡]	No difference in pooled CV events.
VACSDM	153	60	7.8	2.25	2.1%	38%	12%[‡]	Trend for increase in pooled CV events with intensive insulin therapy (p=0.10). Prior CVD major predictor.
DIGAMI	620	68	8	3.4	0.3%	100% (acute MI)	19%[‡] to 26%[†]	29% reduction in 1-year CV mortality with intensive early insulin treatment. 11% absolute reduction in 3.4 years

CV = cardiovascular, CVD = cardiovascular disease, MI = myocardial infarction.
*See text for complete names of studies and references.
[†]CVD deaths.
[‡]Pooled CV events.

study found a HbA1c difference of 7.9 vs. 7.0%. There was a trend toward a reduction in the incidence of myocardial infarction in the intensive management group, but this secondary endpoint did not reach statistical significance. In the Kumamoto Study,[149] cardiovascular event rates were very low in a group of nonobese insulin-sensitive type 2 Japanese diabetics and no difference was seen despite a large HbA1c difference of 2.3% between treatment groups in the 6-year study.

The other two studies gave divergent results. The Veterans Affairs Cooperative Study on Diabetes Mellitus (VACSDM)[3,4] found a trend for an increase in cardiovascular events in intensively treated men who were randomized to a standard vs. intensive insulin treatment policy over a 2.25-year study period. This population was quite different from the UKPDS or Kumamoto patients. The men were elderly, had known diabetes of long duration, had a high prevalence of CVD at baseline, and had a high pooled CV event rate. The best predictor of a CV event in both treatment groups was previous cardiovascular disease. This study suggests that care must be taken if one institutes vigorously intensive glycemic management with insulin in diabetic men who are at high risk for cardiovascular events.

In contrast, the Diabetes Insulin-Glucose in Acute Myocardial Infarction (DIGAMI) study[135,136] has shown that a policy of intensive insulin and supportive management during the course of a myocardial infarction significantly reduces long-term mortality. The trend was seen early and was most significant in patients with mild diabetes, no prior insulin treatment, and less severe damage from myocardial infarction. The mechanism was unclear, but it may be postulated that intensive management had an acute effect on platelet function, fibrinolysis, and/or thrombus formation in patients with an evolving myocardial infarction.

Support for a policy of intensive insulin therapy in critically ill patients (with or without diabetes) is provided by a recent study in critically ill patients admitted to a surgical intensive care unit.[208] Patients were randomly assigned on admission to receive insulin therapy to maintain plasma glucose between 80 and 110 mg/dl, vs. conventional therapy maintaining plasma glucose between 180 and 200 mg/dl. After 1 year, mortality during intensive care was reduced from 8.9% with conventional therapy to 4.6% with intensive therapy in 1548 patients.

It is apparent that additional intervention trials are needed to explore efficacy and safety of intensive glucose management on cardiovascular endpoints in type 2 diabetes. Two large-scale trials—the VA Diabetes Trial and the NHLBI-NIH sponsored Action to Control Cardiovascular Risk in Diabetes (ACCORD) Trial—are now under way to explore this critical issue. Until these studies are finished, we must conclude that, although the evidence favors an intensive glucose management strategy to prevent or delay progression of retinopathy, nephropathy, and neuropathy in type 2 diabetes, its long-term effect on macrovascular endpoints remains open to further study. Intensive insulin management in acutely ill hyperglycemic patients with myocardial infarction or critically ill patients in an intensive care unit is supported by prospective trial data.

Key Points: Evidence for Intensive Glucose Control

- Type 2 diabetes is a progressive disorder, characterized by insulin resistance and insulin deficiency.
- Oral drug therapy may be effectively used, alone or in combination, to address insulin resistance, increased hepatic glucose output, insulin deficiency, and carbohydrate absorption.
- Need for monotherapy, two or more oral agents, and insulin (alone or in combination with oral agent[s]) may generally be predicted by duration of diabetes and prevailing plasma glucose and/or HbA1c levels.
- A perspective on the longitudinal profile of insulin resistance and insulin deficiency in type 2 diabetes provides a useful conceptual framework to guide therapeutic approaches.
- Intensive glucose control has been shown to delay progression of retinopathy and indices of nephropathy and neuropathy in type 2 diabetes.
- Strong epidemiologic data show a correlation between HbA1c and degree of hyperglycemia and cardiovascular events in type 2 diabetes.
- In contrast, long-term prospective trial data of conventional vs. standard glycemic management are conflicting regarding efficacy and safety of intensive management and cardiovascular events.
- Guidelines for intensive glucose management should be more liberal in type 2 diabetics with cardiovascular disease than in those without cardiovascular disease.
- New trials are under way to explore the key issue of long-term intensive glucose control in type 2 diabetes.
- Short-term intensive insulin management of hyperglycemic patients with myocardial infarction or acutely ill patients in a surgical intensive care unit has been shown to significantly reduce mortality compared with standard glycemic management.

Medical Nutrition Therapy

Obesity is characteristic of type 2 diabetes. Depending on the population studied, from 90–95% of people with type 2 diabetes in the U.S. are overweight. Obesity increases the risk for developing diabetes, and the obese diabetic has a markedly increased cardiovascular risk. A classification based on BMI is given in Table 2. Table 3 specifies BMI for various heights and weights. The formula for calculating BMI is weight (lb)/height^2 (in) $\times$ 704.5.

Recent reviews have given evidence about weight management strategies.[134] The best evidence is from well-designed, randomized, controlled trials that provide a constant pattern of findings. These weight management statements are supported by the best scientific evidence:[26]

- All low-calorie diets result in loss of body weight and body fat. Macronutrient composition does not appear to play a major role.
- A moderate-fat weight reduction diet (20–30% calories from fat) is nutritionally adequate.
- Metabolic profiles are improved with energy restriction and weight loss.
- Caloric balance is the major determinant of weight loss. Diets that reduce caloric intake result in weight loss. In the absence of physical activity, the optimal diet for weight loss contains 1,400–1,500 kcal/day, regardless of macronutrient composition.
- Overweight people consuming moderate-fat weight reduction diets lose weight because they consume fewer calories. These diets can produce weight loss when consumed ad libitum.
- Moderate-fat, balanced-nutrient weight reduction diets reduce plasma cholesterol and triglycerides and return the ratio of HDL and total cholesterol toward or to normal.

In type 2 diabetes, the emphasis of medical nutrition therapy is on a meal plan and exercise program that encourage long-term weight reduction. In general, after overall nutrition assessment by a registered dietician, moderate caloric restriction (250–500 calories less than average daily intake from food history) and a modest increase in physical activity (i.e., 30 minutes/day of brisk walking) are prescribed. As little as 5% decrease in weight improves glycemic control and delays progression from IGT to diabetes. Unfortunately, traditional dietary strategies have not been highly successful in maintaining long-term weight loss. It is hoped that more research into how to develop effective lifestyle changes

Table 2. Classification of Weight Categories Based on BMI	
Weight Category	**BMI (kg/m^2)**
Underweight	<18.5
Normal	18.5–24.9
Overweight	25.0–29.9
Obesity	30.0–39.9
Extreme obesity	≥40

Table 3. Body Mass Index Table

BMI	19	20	21	22	23	24	25	26	27	28	29	30	31	32	33	34	35
Height (inches)							Body Weight (pounds)										
58	91	96	100	105	110	115	119	124	129	134	138	143	148	153	158	162	167
59	94	99	104	109	114	119	124	128	133	138	143	148	153	158	163	168	173
60	97	102	107	112	118	123	128	133	138	143	148	153	158	163	168	174	179
61	100	106	111	116	122	127	132	137	143	148	153	158	164	169	174	180	185
62	104	109	115	120	126	131	136	142	147	153	158	164	169	175	180	186	191
63	107	113	118	124	130	135	141	146	152	158	163	169	175	180	186	191	197
64	110	116	122	128	134	140	145	151	157	163	169	174	180	186	192	197	204
65	114	120	126	132	138	144	150	156	162	168	174	180	186	192	198	204	210
66	118	124	130	136	142	148	155	161	167	173	179	186	192	198	204	210	216
67	121	127	134	140	146	153	159	166	172	178	185	191	198	204	211	217	223
68	125	131	138	144	151	158	164	171	177	184	190	197	203	210	216	223	230
69	128	135	142	149	155	162	169	176	182	189	196	203	209	216	223	230	236
70	132	139	146	153	160	167	174	181	188	195	202	209	216	222	229	236	243
71	136	143	150	157	165	172	179	186	193	200	208	215	222	229	236	243	250
72	140	147	154	162	169	177	184	191	199	206	213	221	228	235	242	250	258
73	144	151	159	166	174	182	189	197	204	212	219	227	235	242	250	257	265
74	148	155	163	171	179	186	194	202	210	218	225	233	241	249	256	264	272
75	152	160	168	176	184	192	200	208	216	224	232	240	248	256	264	272	279
76	156	164	172	180	189	197	205	213	221	230	238	246	254	263	271	279	287

(continued)

Table 3. Body Mass Index Table (Continued)

BMI	36	37	38	39	40	41	42	43	44	45	46	47	48	49	50	51	52	53	54
Height (inches)									Body Weight (pound)										
58	172	177	181	186	191	196	201	205	210	215	220	224	229	234	239	244	248	253	258
59	178	183	188	193	198	203	208	212	217	222	227	232	237	242	247	252	257	262	267
60	184	189	194	199	204	209	215	220	225	230	235	240	245	250	255	261	266	271	276
61	190	195	201	206	211	217	222	227	232	238	243	248	254	259	264	269	275	280	285
62	196	202	207	213	218	224	229	235	240	246	251	256	262	267	273	278	284	289	295
63	203	208	214	220	225	231	237	242	248	254	259	265	270	276	282	287	293	299	304
64	209	215	221	227	232	238	244	250	256	262	267	273	279	285	291	296	302	308	314
65	216	222	228	234	240	246	252	258	264	270	276	282	288	294	300	306	312	318	324
66	223	229	235	241	247	253	260	266	272	278	284	291	297	303	309	315	322	328	334
67	230	236	242	249	255	261	268	274	280	287	293	299	306	312	319	325	331	338	344
68	236	243	249	256	262	269	276	282	289	295	302	308	315	322	328	335	341	348	354
69	243	250	257	263	270	277	284	291	297	304	311	318	324	331	338	345	351	358	365
70	250	257	264	271	278	285	292	299	306	313	320	327	334	341	348	355	362	369	376
71	257	265	272	279	286	293	301	308	315	322	329	338	343	351	358	365	372	379	386
72	265	272	279	287	294	302	309	316	324	331	338	346	353	361	368	375	383	390	397
73	272	280	288	295	302	310	318	325	333	340	348	355	363	371	378	386	393	401	408
74	280	287	295	303	311	319	326	334	342	350	358	365	373	381	389	396	404	412	420
75	287	295	303	311	319	327	335	343	351	359	367	375	383	391	399	407	415	423	431
76	295	304	312	320	328	336	344	353	361	369	377	385	394	402	410	418	426	435	443

From Bessen DH, Kushner R: Evaluation and Management of Obesity. Philadelphia, Hanley & Belfus, 2002, p 11, with permission.

regarding eating and physical activity will improve this situation in the future.

In the meantime, it is appropriate to review the goals and objectives of medical nutrition therapy in type 2 diabetes. It is also important to give current recommendations for meal and exercise planning, as well as distribution of calories as carbohydrate, protein, and fat and to discuss such special issues as types of carbohydrate and fat, alcohol, fiber, and micronutrients in medical nutrition therapy.[11]

Goals of Medical Nutrition Therapy

The overall goal is to assist the type 2 diabetic in developing an individualized nutrition and exercise plan that will help lead to optimal metabolic control.[11] Thus, the plan should achieve nearly normal blood glucose and HbA1c levels, and optimal plasma lipid concentrations, provide adequate calories for maintaining or achieving reasonable weight, and improve overall health through optimal nutrition. Medical nutrition therapy must also consider special issues such as hypoglycemia, renal or congestive heart failure, hypertension, dyslipidemia, and the actions of therapeutic agents for diabetes and its complications.

Calorie Distribution

Although medical nutrition therapy has been recognized historically as the cornerstone of long-term management of people with type 2 diabetes, recommendations for distribution of carbohydrates, protein, and fat in the diet have had remarkable shifts in emphasis (Table 4).

After many years of recommending relatively high-fat diets in diabetes, there was a gradual shift to individualized nutritional recommendations, with particular emphasis on dropping the percentage of calories as fat in view of the relationship between saturated fat intake and atherosclerosis. The most recent recommendations for calorie distribution from the American Diabetes Association are as follows: carbohydrates and monounsaturated fats should provide 60–70% of total caloric intake; protein intake, 15–20%; total fat, <30%; saturated fat, <10%.

Table 4. Distribution of Calories (%)			
Year	Carbohydrate	Protein	Fat
1950	40	20	40
1971	45	20	35
1986	≤ 60	12–20	<30
1994	*	10–20*†	*†

*Based on nutritional assessment and treatment goals.
†Less than 10% of calories from saturated fat.

Carbohydrates

Sucrose or sucrose-containing foods are no longer banned in the dietary prescription. They must be calculated as part of the total carbohydrate prescription rather than adding them to the plan. Dietary fructose, as contained in many fruits and some vegetables, is acceptable except in type 2 diabetics with dyslipidemia characterized by high plasma triglyceride and low HDL cholesterol levels. Some physicians and dieticians favor an approach that emphasizes foods with low glycemic indices to decrease postprandial glycemic excursions. However, long-term studies of this approach have not yielded definitive results. The nonnutritive sweeteners (aspartame, saccharin) may be used and have no caloric impact.

Protein

In the absence of solid scientific data to establish precisely optimal protein intake in uncomplicated type 2 diabetes, the recommendations have remained fairly stable over the years.

In one study of obese type 2 diabetics,[153] a high protein weight loss diet (30% protein, 42% carbohydrate, 28% fat) was associated with reduction in LDL cholesterol and in total and abdominal fat mass in women compared with a lower protein weight loss diet (15% protein, 60% carbohydrate, 25% fat). The authors concluded that this was a valid diet choice for reducing cardiovascular risk in type 2 diabetes. It is clear that more research is needed to guide nutrition therapy in type 2 diabetes.

Although the large-scale trial data are not convincing, most physicians and nutritionists recommend protein restriction in the presence of renal failure. Early in nephropathy, with albuminuria and nearly normal plasma creatinine levels, 0.8 gm/kg/day of protein is recommended. If the glomerular filtration rate falls, further restriction to 0.6–0.7 gm/kg/day may be associated with lower plasma urea nitrogen levels.

Fat

There appears to be general agreement that total dietary fat should be less than 30% of prescribed calories. Cholesterol intake should be less than 300 mg/day. Fat restriction is an efficient way to lower calorie consumption, because each gram of fat contains 9 calories, whereas one gram of carbohydrate or protein contains 4 calories. Distribution of fat should be about 10–15% as polyunsaturated and 10–15% of monounsaturated fat, unless dyslipidemia is present. In that case, a higher percentage (15–20%) of monounsaturated fat is indicated, and fat calories should be exchanged for carbohydrate calories. The use of unsaturated fat of the omega-3 variety (fish oils, flaxseed or mustard oil) is becoming a popular approach, with about 3 gm/day as the recommendation.

Controlled short-term studies have shown that high doses (usually at least 3 gm/day) of omega-3 fatty acids significantly lower plasma triglyceride levels in type 2 diabetes. Thus, in type 2 patients with dyslipidemia characterized by high plasma triglyceride levels, increasing the dietary intake of monounsaturated fatty acids and/or omega-3 fatty acids may be a useful strategy. A concern, however, is that the higher fat diet may contribute to weight gain unless carbohydrate intake is decreased proportionally.

Alcohol

Recent research gives good news to people who enjoy an occasional alcoholic beverage. Three recent epidemiologic studies have examined the association between alcohol consumption and the risk of coronary heart disease in people with type 2 diabetes.[6,187,207] Risk reductions for coronary heart disease of 34–79% were associated with light-to-moderate alcohol intake. Studies in people without diabetes have been confirmatory, with over 40 studies showing a reduction in CHD risk of 10–40% associated with alcohol intake of 1–3 drinks per day. The benefits apply to alcoholic drinks of all types, not just wine. A summary of the three critical cohort studies in type 2 diabetes is given in Table 5.

Prospective randomized trials are needed to explore this issue directly. In the meantime, recommendations are no more than 2 drinks per day for men and 1 per day for women. Because of alcohol's inhibition of glucose production by hepatic gluconeogenesis in the fasting state, food should be taken with alcohol. One alcoholic beverage is substituted for 2 fat exchanges to keep total calories constant.

Table 5. Prospective Studies on Alcohol Intake and CHD in Type 2 Diabetes					
Author	Study Name	Type 2 DM	Follow-up (yr)	CHD Events	RR
Valmadrid	Wisconsin Epidemiologic Study of Diabetes Retinopathy	444 M 539 F	12	198 CHD deaths	0.21
Solomon	Nurses' Health Study	5103 F	14	295 Events Nonfatal MI Fatal CHD	0.47 0.43
Ajani	Physicians' Health Study	2790 M (enrollment) 5074 M (randomized)	5.5 12	133 CHD deaths 120 events (MI/CABG)	0.42 0.66
CABG = Coronary artery bypass graft, CHD = coronary heart disease, MI = myocardial infarction, RR = relative risk for moderate alcohol vs. no alcohol drinking. (References for the studies are given in the text.)					

Other Issues

Dietary fiber of the soluble type may help to lower plasma lipid levels. Recommendations for total fiber intake parallel those for the general population: 20–35 gm/day of both soluble and insoluble fibers. The rationale for this recommendation also includes possible beneficial effects of high fiber intake on constipation and colon cancer. Furthermore, fiber may provide increased satiety and thereby help with weight reduction diets.

In general, vitamin or mineral supplementation is recommended only if dietary intake or loss of nutrients due to disease (e.g., prolonged glycosuria) is present. Chromium replacement may have a beneficial effect on glucose control in the presence of chromium deficiency. Similarly, in patients with evidence of magnesium or potassium depletion, supplementation is indicated. Moderate sodium restriction (≤ 2.4 gm/day) is recommended for hypertension and ≤ 2.0 gm/day for hypertension and nephropathy.

In summary, for most people with type 2 diabetes, the goal is to achieve a metabolic state in which calorie intake is less than caloric expenditure. This is the real challenge of medical nutrition therapy in type 2 diabetes—and one that is desperately in need of improved strategies to achieve long-term weight reduction. A promising development was the announcement that beginning on January 1, 2002, medical nutrition therapy is covered by Medicare when provided by a qualifying registered dietician or nutrition professional.

Key Points: Medical Nutrition Therapy

- ⋙ Because obesity and type 2 diabetes are increasing at alarming rates in the U.S., it is apparent that current programs of medical nutrition therapy and exercise are generally not successful.
- ⋙ A major challenge is to develop lifestyle changes of eating and physical activity that produce long-term weight reduction and increased physical fitness among type 2 diabetics.
- ⋙ Goals of medical nutrition and exercise programs are improved physical fitness, reasonable weight control, and optimal metabolic and blood pressure control.
- ⋙ Because weight reduction is a major goal for 90% of people with type 2 diabetes, there is no mystery about meals and exercise. Calories expended each day must exceed those ingested.
- ⋙ An individualized meal plan should be developed with 30% or less as fat, 10–20% as protein, and the remainder as carbohydrate.
- ⋙ There are three useful facts about dietary fat:

Key Points (*Continued*)

1. The ratio of polyunsaturated to monounsaturated fat should be 1:1. Monounsaturated fat is increased and replaces carbohydrate calories if hypertriglyceridemia is a problem.
2. Omega-3 fatty acids may be a useful source of monounsaturated fat.
3. Cholesterol intake should be 300 mg/day or, less.

☞ The good news is that three controlled studies in type 2 diabetic patients have shown that CHD risk reductions of 34–79% were associated with moderate alcohol intake.

☞ Medical nutrition therapy is covered by Medicare when provided by qualified professionals.

Exercise in Type 2 Diabetes

As noted in the chapters on type 1 diabetes, acute exercise may result in lowering blood glucose to hypoglycemic levels. The same effect may also occur in well-controlled type 2 diabetic patients, whether metabolic control has been maintained with an oral agent, combinations of oral agents, or insulin alone or in combination with oral agent(s). However, if metabolic control is not good to excellent, acute exercise may be followed by a rise in blood glucose secondary to increased hepatic glucose production. It is therefore important for the type 2 diabetic to check blood glucose before and immediately after acute exercise on several occasions to determine individual patterns of response.

Regular exercise usually improves overall glucose control in people with type 2 diabetes,[9] as is manifested by a pattern of lower average blood glucose concentrations and a lower HbA1c value, with minimal effect on fasting blood glucose levels. The mechanism is an improvement in insulin sensitivity. This effect, however, is rapidly lost when acute exercise is discontinued but may persist longer (up to 1 week) in physically conditioned patients.

A meta-analysis of 14 clinical trials of aerobic or resistance training of at least 8 weeks in duration in patients with type 2 diabetes has been reported.[27] A significant fall in HbA1c to 7.65% occurred in the exercise groups compared with 8.31% in controls. The effect was independent of weight loss and was seen in middle-aged patients with diverse ethnic backgrounds. The 0.66% reduction in HbA1c, if sustained, would be expected to reduce the risk of microvascular complications.

Many people with type 2 diabetes are at risk for complications from an exercise program. A complete history, physical examination, and critical laboratory tests (e.g., an exercise stress test) are recommended for type 2 diabetics before starting an exercise program. Coronary artery disease may benefit from a supervised exercise program, such as cardiac rehabilitation. Type 2 diabetic patients with proliferative retinopathy may have retinal or vitreous hemorrhage, especially with Valsalva-type maneuvers. Patients with albuminuria may have a transient increase after exercise; but this does not appear to affect progression of renal disease. If peripheral sensory neuropathy is present, damage to soft tissues and/or joints may occur with weight-bearing exercise. Table 6 lists exercises that are contraindicated or recommended for type 2 diabetics individuals with diminution or loss of peripheral sensation.[9] Thus, the exercise prescription must be tailored to the individual patient, depending on the presence or absence of macrovascular or microvascular complications.

Generally, an exercise program should consist of moderately intense aerobic exercises for 30 minutes or more, preferably for 5–7 days each week. Warm-up and cool-down periods of 5–10 minutes each are recommended. In the absence of proliferative retinopathy or uncontrolled hypertension, resistance training and/or high-intensity exercises are useful aids to physical conditioning.

In summary, one of the most promising areas in management of type 2 diabetes has been the increasing interest in physical fitness, especially among adults, in the U.S. It is clear that exercise leading to improved physical fitness is a critical component of overall medical therapy for people with type 2 diabetes.

Table 6. Exercises for People with Peripheral Sensory Neuropathy	
Contraindicated	Recommended
Treadmill	Swimming
Prolonged walking	Bicycling
Jogging	Rowing
Step exercises	Chair or arm exercises

Key Points: Exercise in Type 2 Diabetes

- People with type 2 diabetes should regularly check blood glucose before and immediately after exercise to learn the pattern of change and to predict future management.
- Regular exercise usually improves overall glucose control in type 2 diabetes. The effect is seen in prevailing glucose levels during the day or in HbA1c levels. It is less apparent when fasting blood glucose values are examined.
- The mechanism of improved glucose control is increased insulin sensitivity. This effect is quickly reversed after acute aerobic exercise but may be sustained after prolonged physical conditioning.

Key Points (*Continued*)

⧉ Because patients with type 2 diabetes have an increased cardiovascular risk, a complete cardiovascular assessment, usually including an exercise stress test, should be done before prescribing an exercise program.

⧉ Patients with peripheral sensory neuropathy should choose swimming, bicycling, or rowing rather than weight-bearing exercises such as walking, jogging, treadmill or step exercising.

⧉ Valsalva maneuvers may exacerbate proliferative diabetic retinopathy.

⧉ Optimally, an exercise program should consist of moderately intense aerobic exercise for 30 minutes or more on 5–7 days each week.

Oral Antihyperglycemic Agent Therapy

Oral agents addressing multiple defects that may be present at various stages of type 2 diabetes are now available. Thus, one may choose an agent that stimulates the pancreatic beta cell to immediately release insulin, to release insulin more slowly, to inhibit the breakdown of complex carbohydrates in the gastrointestinal tract, to inhibit hepatic glucose output, or to increase the sensitivity of adipose tissue and muscle to the action of insulin. Because the major pathophysiology of type 2 diabetes is a combination of diminished insulin supply and increased resistance to insulin action, combinations of these agents theoretically should be quite effective in returning glucose metabolism nearly to normal.[100,128]

Table 7 lists selected agents now available in the United States. The range of usual daily dosages is given, as are major sites of action. This section considers their effectiveness and side effects, either as monotherapy or in combination, and concludes with a recommended approach to therapy of type 2 diabetes with oral agents.

Mechanisms of Action

Acute Insulin Secretagogues (Meglitinides)

The meglitinides stimulate the immediate release of insulin by functioning beta cells.[127] They interact with the adenosine triphosphate (ATP)-sensitive potassium (K + ATP) channel to cause depolarization,[97,98] which is followed by calcium influx and by insulin secretion. The extent of insulin release is glucose-dependent and diminishes at low glucose levels or when pancreatic insulin stores are low. Repaglinide, a drug of the meglitinide class, is a benzoic acid derivative.[81] Nateglinide is a phenylalanine derivative.[86] Thus, these two oral agents are not sulfonylureas. Both are rapidly absorbed and act to stimulate immediate insulin release with meals.[110] Duration of action is short. These agents should be

Table 7. Selected Oral Antihyperglycemic Agents		
Agent	**Dose (mg/day)**	**Major Site of Action**
Acute insulin secretagogues (meglitinides)		
Repaglinide	0.5–4 (ac)	Pancreatic beta cell
Nateglinide	60–120 (ac)	Pancreatic beta cell
Acute and chronic insulin secretagogues (sulfonylureas)		
Glipizide	2.5–5 (ac)	Pancreatic beta cell
Glipizide XL	5–10	Pancreatic beta cell
Glyburide	1.25–15	Pancreatic beta cell
Glimepiride	1–8	Pancreatic beta cell
Alpha glucosidase inhibitors		
Acarbose	25–100 (ac)	Intestinal cell
Miglitol	50–100 (ac)	Intestinal cell
Hepatic glucose production inhibitor (biguanide)		
Metformin	500–1000 (bid)*	Liver
Insulin sensitizers (thiazolidinediones)		
Pioglitazone	15–45	Fat, muscle
Rosiglitazone	4–8	Fat, muscle

(ac) = just before meal.
*Take on a full stomach.

given with each meal and act to decrease meal-related glucose excursions in responsive patients.[106]

Acute and Chronic Insulin Secretagogues (Sulfonylureas)

The sulfonylureas are also stimulators of insulin secretion and act through the K+ATP channels of the pancreatic beta cells.[127,128] They have a relatively slow onset of action, and the longer-acting agents (glyburide, glipizide XL, glimeperide) have a prolonged effect on insulin secretion. These agents have less of an effect on immediate insulin release than the acute insulin secretagogues and may be taken once or twice daily. Glipizide is more rapid-acting and appears to be most effective if taken 2 or 3 times daily with meals. Glipizide XL is a longer-acting preparation designed to be taken once daily.

Alpha-Glucosidase Inhibitors

Acarbose and miglitol are inhibitors of the enzymes that break down dietary starch. Complex carbohydrates in the diet are broken down to oligosaccharides by pancreatic amylase. The α-glucosidase enzymes break down oligosaccharides into monosaccharides in the duodenum and upper jejunum. Acarbose and miglitol are competitive inhibitors of the binding of oligosaccharides to the enzymes. The net result is a slow absorption of dietary carbohydrate and a decrease in the postprandial glucose response.[125,127,128] Glycemic control may improve.

Hepatic Glucose Production Inhibitor (Biguanide)

Metformin is a biguanide, a class of drugs that has long been recognized to have antihyperglycemic actions.[17,18] In medieval times, it was reported that *Galega officinalis* (goat's rue or French lilac) was used for treatment of diabetes in Europe. This plant was rich in guanidine, which has hypoglycemic activity. Various derivatives (galegine, synthalin) were found to be hepatotoxic in clinical trials. A guanidine derivative, phenformin, was removed from the U.S. market in 1975 because of lactic acidosis. Thus, the history of these agents was not promising and probably contributed to the rather late submission and approval by the FDA of metformin for use in the United States in 1994, after it had been available for use in Europe and Canada for many years.[44]

Early studies suggested that the major mechanism of action of metformin in type 2 diabetes was an increase in insulin-stimulated glucose uptake by skeletal muscle. More recently, it has been shown that metformin acts primarily by inhibiting hepatic glucose output and decreasing both gluconeogenesis and glycogenolysis.[51] The increased insulin sensitivity seen in previous studies may have been due to decreased glucose toxicity. Metformin also decreases appetite, and long-term use is not associated with the weight gain that usually accompanies improved glycemic control with other agents in type 2 diabetes.[30,100,101]

Insulin Sensitizers (Thiazolidinediones)

Pioglitazone and rosiglitazone are two new agents of the thiazolidinedione class that decrease insulin resistance.[126,143] The first agent of this class to be introduced was troglitazone, which was removed from the U.S. market by the FDA because of liver toxicity.[213] These drugs act on the peroxisome proliferator-activated receptor (PPAR) family of nuclear receptors. A subtype, PPAR γ, is activated by the thiazolidinediones and acts on genes with protein products that regulate lipid metabolism and insulin action. The precise mechanism by which PPAR γ agonists improve insulin sensitivity is not known. The primary action may be on muscle or on fat. Free fatty acid levels fall. Intraabdominal fat mass decreases, and the larger subcutaneous adipose cells proliferate into smaller, more insulin-sensitive cells. Overall, the major effect of thiazolidenediones on insulin action is to increase insulin-mediated glucose uptake by muscle.[126,128,143]

Effectiveness of Oral Agents

Monotherapy

Therapy with one oral agent is usually the first step when a type 2 diabetic patient has failed to meet glycemic control guidelines (HbA1c

<7%) after a period of therapy by medical nutrition and exercise. Monotherapy may be used more frequently in prediabetic patients with IGT or IFG in the future. The Diabetes Prevention Program[52] conclusively showed that monotherapy may delay or prevent the onset of diabetes in patients with impaired glucose tolerance and normal HbA1c levels. Several fundamental facts have emerged from controlled studies with one oral agent in people with type 2 diabetes:[100,128]

- Newly diagnosed (drug-naive) diabetics respond better to single-agent therapy than longstanding diabetic patients.
- Compared with placebo, monotherapy of drug-naive patients with sulfonylureas, metformin, or thiazolidinediones usually results in a drop in hemoglobin A1c of 1.5–2.0%.
- The effects of the acute insulin stimulators (repaglinide, nateglinide) and alpha gucosidase inhibitors (acarbose, miglitol) are primarily on postprandial glucose levels. Their effects on HbA1c values are usually in the range of 0.5–1.0% in drug-naive patients.
- None of the agents, when used as monotherapy, chronically lowers HbA1c below 7% in the majority of patients.
- Because of this fact and because type 2 diabetes is a progressive disease, therapy with multiple agents and/or insulin is usually needed with increasing duration of type 2 diabetes.[201]
- In the UKPDS, metformin monotherapy significantly reduced the incidence of myocardial infarction (39%) and diabetes-related deaths (32%) in overweight type 2 diabetics.[203] This effect was not seen with insulin or sulfonylurea therapy despite similar HbA1c changes. For this reason and because weight gain is usually not seen with metformin, many physicians choose this biguanide as the first choice for monotherapy in drug-naive overweight type 2 diabetic patients with good renal function.

Combined Oral Agent Therapy

Two Agents

Various combination therapy approaches with the oral agents have been studied. As reviewed by Lebovitz,[128] FDA registration studies are summarized in Table 8. Several points are apparent from these studies:

1. The second agent must be added to the first, not substituted for it.
2. Maximal doses of both drugs are generally reported in the table.
3. Glycemic regulation, as judged by mean HbA1c >8%, was at the ADA-recommended action level in the majority of studies. Thus, monotherapy was not effective in meeting guidelines.
4. HbA1c decreases of 0.7–2.2% were seen, but the majority were in the 0.7–1.4% range.

5. Very few oral drug combinations were effective in reaching a HbA1c goal of ≤ 7%.
6. Although differences from placebo are not shown in this table, conclusions are comparable when placebo results are reviewed.

More Than Two Oral Agents

Because oral antihyperglycemic agents have different modes of action and because dual oral agent therapy may not reduce HbA1c levels to the desired goal, it is reasonable to consider the addition of a third agent. This option became realistic when the thiazolidinediones and the immediate insulin stimulators became available. There are few controlled studies of this approach; in addition, the removal of troglitazone from the market seriously limited interpretation of available studies with thiazolidinedione as the third agent. In one prospective, randomized, placebo-controlled trial, 200 patients receiving maximal doses of sulfonylureas and metformin were randomly assigned to the addition of troglitazone (400 mg/day) or placebo.[216] The triple-therapy group had a fall in HbA1c of 1.2% vs an increase of 0.2% in the placebo group. Forty-three percent of the triple-therapy group achieved HbA1c <8% vs. 6% on placebo. There was a 2.9-kg weight gain in the triple-therapy group. More studies are needed to evaluate fully the benefits and risks of triple therapy, particularly with long-term use. Such studies are now under way.

			Additional	Percentage
Drug	**Dose (mg/day)**	**Baseline mean HbA1c(%)**	**decrease in HbA1c(%)**	**attaining HbA1c ≤ 7%**
Metformin ≥ 2000 mg/day+				
Glyburide	20	8.8	1.3	NA
Repaglinide	12	8.3	1.1	~60
Nateglinide	360	8.4	0.7	NA
Acarbose	600	7.8	0.8	NA
Rosiglitazone	8	8.9	1.2	28
Pioglitazone	30	9.9	0.8	NA
Rosiglitazone 8 mg/day+				
Repaglinide	12	9.2	1.15	NA
Sulfonylurea			1.4	NA
Pioglitazone 30 mg/day+				
Repaglinide	12	9.6	2.2	NA
Sulfonylurea	*	10.0	1.3	NA

Table 8. Effect of Combination Therapy with Oral Antihyperglycemic Agents on Glycemic Control in FDA Registration Studies

NA = not available.
*Dose depends on agent used

Key Points: Oral Agent Therapy

∞ Oral agents are now available to address the key pathophysiologic issues in type 2 diabetes: decreased insulin secretion, increased insulin resistance, and increased hepatic glucose production
∞ Either sulfonylureas or meglitinides may be used to stimulate insulin secretion.
∞ The thiazolidinediones and metformin act as insulin sensitizers.
∞ Metformin's major mechanism of action is to decrease hepatic glucose output.
∞ Monotherapy with these agents generally lowers HbA1c 1–2% in newly diagnosed type 2 diabetic patients.
∞ Metformin is the drug of first choice in recently diagnosed overweight type 2 diabetic patients who have HbA1c values > 7% despite diet and exercise lifestyle programs.
∞ Addition of a second agent is usually needed to achieve therapeutic goals, particularly in people with diabetes of 5–10 years' duration.
∞ A stimulator of insulin secretion (meglitinide or sulfonylurea) is added as the second agent if metformin monotherapy fails to reach HbA1c goals.
∞ Other combinations may be tried empirically before insulin is added.
∞ Insulin in combination with oral agent(s) is usually needed as type 2 diabetes increases in duration.

Side Effects of Oral Agent Therapy

Acute Insulin Secretagogues (Meglitinides)

Because repaglinide and nateglinide stimulate acute insulin release by a responsive pancreas, hypoglycemia may occur with either agent. For this reason the agents should be given immediately before food ingestion. In such cases, hypoglycemia is rare, and if it occurs, the dosage of the agent should be decreased. These drugs appear to be most effective in the early stages of type 2 diabetes (Fig. 2, Chapter 8), when pancreatic insulin stores and responsive beta cells are still present. The frequency of hypoglycemia is similar to that seen with short-acting sulfonylureas (e.g., glipizide).

The liver is the main site of metabolism of repaglinide and nateglinide, and both agents should be used with caution in the presence of liver injury. Both drugs are metabolized primarily by the cytochrome P-350 hepatic enzyme system, and in vitro data indicate that repaglinide metabolism may be inhibited by antifungal agents (e.g., ketoconazole) and erythromycin. Drug interactions have been studied with both agents; interaction with commonly used drugs to date appear to be of no clinical significance.

Weight gain is usually seen when type 2 diabetes is controlled with insulin-secretagogues, primarily because of retention of calories that previously were lost through glycosuria (100 grams of glucose in the urine = 400 calories). Few long-term studies with the acute insulin secretagogues have addressed weight gain.

Acute and Chronic Insulin Secretagogues (Sulfonylureas)

Most of the sulfonylureas in current use are metabolized by the liver and excreted by the kidney. Thus, they must be used with caution, or not at all, in the presence of hepatic disease or renal insufficiency. Because glipizide's hepatic metabolites are inactive, it theoretically may have an advantage in renal insufficiency. Because glimepiride's active metabolite is cleared by the liver, it also has a theoretical advantage in the presence of renal insufficiency.

Severe hypoglycemia may occur with the sulfonylureas and is usually seen in older people with newly diagnosed type 2 diabetes or when the drugs are used in the presence of renal insufficiency. Glyburide is the most common offender. In several large clinical studies, serious hypoglycemia was reported in 1.4–1.7% of patients per year with glyburide therapy. Deaths from hypoglycemia have been reported with glyburide therapy. Glipizide and glimepiride have significantly lower rates of serious hypoglycemia than glyburide.

Weight gain is often seen with long-term sulfonylurea therapy. Glyburide treatment is accompanied by a 2- to 4-kg weight gain after 1–2 years of treatment. In the UKPDS, a weight gain of about 3 kg occurred in the sulfonylurea-treated overweight patients. Most of the weight gain occurred in the first 2–3 years and was seen even though HbA1c levels were increasing. Thus, the precise reasons for weight gain with long-term sulfonylurea therapy are not completely understood.[101]

Controversy has continued since the University Group Diabetes Program (UGDP) report of increased cardiovascular mortality in patients randomized to tolbutamide vs. insulin or diet alone.[2] These findings have not been confirmed by any subsequent randomized controlled trial. In particular, there was no evidence of cardiac toxicity in patients randomized to sulfonylurea therapy in the UKPDS, compared with insulin or diet alone.[205] There was a trend toward a decrease in the secondary endpoint of myocardial infarction in the group randomized to intensive therapy with oral agents and/or insulin compared with the group assigned to a less intensive glycemic control policy.

Other adverse effects include skin rashes, which occur in approximately

1% or less of patients. The sulfonylureas should not be used in patients with sulfa drug sensitivity.

Alpha Glucosidase Inhibitors (Acarbose, Miglitol)

Gastrointestinal side effects are frequent. Breakdown of carbohydrates is limited by drug action, and the increased delivery of carbohydrates to the colon results in gas production by fermentation. As many as 60–70% of patients report flatulence with acarbose or miglitol therapy. Occasionally, cramps and/or diarrhea may be present. To minimize these side effects, it is important to start with very low doses of the drug (i.e., 25 mg with the evening meal) and to increase the frequency and dosage slowly over weeks or months, as tolerated. Because of the gastrointestinal side effects, they should not be used in patients with symptomatic bowel disease. Hypoglycemia is not a side effect of this class of drugs. However, if they are used in combination with insulin or insulin secretagogues, hypoglycemia can occur. In this case, glucose should be used for treatment of the low blood glucose, because the alpha glucosidase inhibitor will inhibit the breakdown of more complex carbohydrates to glucose. Elevation of hepatic enzymes was reported in a few patients when high doses (100 mg 3 times/day) of acarbose were used in older studies. This has not been a serious problem under the lower dose schedules now recommended.

Inhibitor of Hepatic Glucose Output (Metformin)

Metformin's major side effects are also gastrointestinal. They usually consist of abdominal discomfort or diarrhea, and may occur in up to 30% of patients. These side effects are dose-related and can be minimized by taking the lowest effective doses when the stomach is full. They are also less when the patient starts with a low dose (500 mg) with the evening meal, and then works up to the final effective dose with breakfast and supper. With time, most patients tolerate a schedule or either 500 mg with each of 3 meals or 1.0 gm with breakfast and supper to achieve maximal blood glucose effect. A small percentage of patients (< 10%) cannot continue to take the drug because of side effects.

Lactic acidosis with metformin therapy is a rare complication in contrast to the earlier biguanide, phenformin. It is reported in only 3.3 cases/100,000 person years and is virtually absent if proper contraindications are observed. Because metformin is excreted by the kidneys as the parent compound, blood levels may rise in the presence of renal insufficiency. Thus, the drug is contraindicated if the serum creatinine level is above the normal range. Because hypoxemia may contribute to lactic acidosis, metformin should not be used in hypoxic states, such as may occur with congestive heart failure, severe pulmonary disease, or severe illnesses associated with hypotension and poor organ perfusion. It is also contraindicated in alcoholism or active liver disease. The drug should be discontinued if a patient undergoes an intravenous dye study or major surgery, withheld for 48 hours, and restarted only if serum creatinine levels are in the normal range.

Finally, low serum vitamin B_{12} levels may occur with metformin therapy because of an inference with absorption. Anemia appears to be rare.

Insulin Sensitizers (Thiazolidinediones)

The first thiazolidinedione to be approved for clinical use in the U.S. was troglitazone. It has now been withdrawn from the market by the FDA because of liver toxicity,[213] which was manifested by hepatic failure and death in a small number of patients and by elevations of hepatic enzymes in others. In clinical trials, 1.9% of patients treated with troglitazone developed hepatic enzyme levels three times the upper limit of normal (or more) compared with 0.6% of placebo-treated patients. In contrast, neither pioglitazone nor rosiglitazone showed evidence of liver toxicity compared with placebo in clinical trials. Because of the troglitazone experience, liver function tests are recommended before starting therapy with rosiglitazone or pioglitazone and periodically thereafter. Therapy should not be started in patients with clinical evidence of active liver disease or alanine aminotransferase (ALT) levels that exceed 2.5 times the upper limit of normal. Clinical experience over about 2 years of experience with these two agents has not indicated that there is an undue risk of liver toxicity.[100,128]

A major problem is that these drugs are often associated with fluid retention and peripheral edema. An expanded plasma volume and a fall in hematocrit may be noted. Congestive heart failure may occur, particularly when insulin is also used, and the drugs are contraindicated in patients with New York Heart Association class III or IV heart failure. Package labeling addresses this issue. The mechanism for fluid retention is under study. Weight gain is usually in the range of 2–3 kg/year with monotherapy and reaches 4–5 kg with combined therapy with insulin or sulfonylureas. This excessive weight is due partially to fluid retention and partially to proliferation of subcutaneous adipose tissue cells. Some of the weight gain is presumably the same phenomenon seen with improved glycemic control with insulin and sulfonylureas, alone or in combination. However, further study of the precise reasons for weight gain is indicated.[143]

On the other hand, the thiazolidinediones are associated with changes in cardiovascular risk factors that may be beneficial in patients with metabolic syndrome or type 2 diabetes.[154] Such changes include the following:

- Fall in blood pressure[154]
- Improvement in diabetic dyslipidemia[173]

- Decrease in microalbuminuria[20,99]
- Decrease in carotid intima-medial thickness[115,140]
- Lowering of elevated plasma PAI-1 levels[62]
- In vitro and animal studies suggesting antiatherogenic actions[39,74,124]

Overview of Oral Agent Therapy

The perspective on the management of type 2 diabetes given in Figure 2, Chapter 8, is based on the usual progression from a stage of impaired glucose tolerance to gradually more serious metabolic decompensation with increasing duration of diabetes. At early stages, if a nutrition and exercise plan fails to lower HbA1c below 7%, a single oral agent is recommended. In overweight type 2 diabetic patients, most physicians favor metformin as the first drug based on three main facts: (1) efficacy is about the same as other drugs; (2) weight gain is less likely to occur; and (3) in the UKPDS, metformin as the initial therapy was associated with a significant decrease in myocardial infarction and cardiovascular deaths compared with oral sulfonylurea, insulin, or diet therapy.[203] In nonobese type 2 diabetics, it seems reasonable to start with a drug to stimulate the sluggish first-phase insulin secretion—a meglitinide or a sulfonylurea.

As time progresses, during the first 10 years or so of type 2 diabetes, monotherapy often fails to reach glycemic targets, and a second agent is needed. Action is indicated when HbA1c is > 8%, and the goal is HbA1c < 7%. In this phase (II or III in Fig. 2, Chapter 8), a sulfonylurea is added to metformin (and vice versa in nonobese patients). Failure to reach the goal can lead to other combinations (e.g., meglitinide plus thiazolidinedione, or metformin or sulfonylurea plus thiazolidinedione). An alpha glucosidase inhibitor may be used in low doses as an ancillary third drug with any of these combinations. It is important to recognize the requirement for multiple therapies in most type 2 diabetic patients as the disease progresses.[201]

Long-term studies of triple or quadruple (or more) oral drug therapy are limited in number. Therefore, most physicians start insulin therapy, in combination with oral drug therapy, if the combinations of two oral drugs do not maintain HbA1c below 8%. Insulin in combination with oral drugs or insulin therapy alone are discussed in the following section.

Key Points: Side Effects of Oral Agent Therapy

☞ Acute stimulators of insulin release (meglitinides) may produce hypoglycemia if the dosage is too high for the ingested meal or if the drug is taken without a meal.

☞ If hepatic injury is present, the majority of oral agents are either contraindicated or must be used with caution.

Key Points (*Continued*)

⤷ Glyburide involves the greatest risk of severe hypoglycemia, particularly with renal insufficiency and in older patients.

⤷ Weight gain is a side effect of successful glycemic therapy with all oral agents except metformin.

⤷ Although an older study (UGDP)[2] indicated an increased cardiovascular risk associated with sulfonylurea therapy, this finding has not been confirmed in a modern study (UKPDS).[205]

⤷ The alpha glucosidase inhibitors are best used as ancillary agents because of gastrointestinal side effects and low efficacy.

⤷ Metformin's major side effects are gastrointestinal, but they are limited by titrating dosage upward and taking divided doses on a full stomach.

⤷ Lactic acidosis is rare with metformin, but the drug should not be used in patients with elevated serum creatinine levels or hypoxic states or when radiographic contrast media is used.

⤷ The thiazolidinediones usually cause weight gain, some of which is attributed to fluid retention.

⤷ Thiazolidinediones are contraindicated in patients with New York Heart Association class III or IV heart failure and may precipitate congestive heart failure in other patients.

⤷ Thiazolidinediones and meglitinides may be used in the presence of renal insufficiency in contrast to sulfonylureas and metformin.

Insulin Therapy

Combination Therapy: Oral Agents and Insulin

Rationale

As type 2 diabetes progresses, many patients do not achieve currently recommended glycemic goals on single doses of oral agents, despite repetitive attempts at nutrition planning and exercise programs. In the UKPDS, for instance, only 50% of patients obtained a HbA1c goal of < 7% after 3 years of oral agent monotherapy, and this figure dropped to 25% after 9 years.[201,205,215] Before the introduction of meglitinides, metformin, and thiazolidinediones, 43% of people with type 2 diabetes in the U.S. required insulin therapy. Insulin use increased to 58% of patients with diabetes of ≥ 20 years' duration. Such patients usually have depleted beta cell reserves and increasing insulin resistance secondary to prolonged hyperglycemia ("glucose toxicity"). Large insulin doses (≥1 U/kg) are often necessary to achieve excellent glycemic control in such patients, even under carefully controlled conditions. Because of some concern that these large doses may be harmful to the vascular system, and because such doses of insulin often are associated with weight gain (or an inability to lose weight), most physicians now favor combining oral agent therapy with evening insulin[165,166,167] in attempts to reach the recommended HbA1c goal of < 7%. A thorough discussion of insulin therapy in type 2 diabetes is available elsewhere.[142]

Sulfonylureas and Bedtime Insulin

A combination of a sulfonylurea with bedtime insulin is often effective.[166,167] One large prospective study that explored this issue in a controlled way is the Veterans Affairs Cooperative Study on Diabetes Mellitus,[4,5] in which 153 adult men with longstanding type 2 diabetes were randomly assigned to standard insulin therapy or an intensive glycemic management strategy in which four steps were followed with a HbA1c level of <7.0% as the goal. These steps were as follows: (1) bedtime NPH insulin was increased in dosage to achieve a morning fasting plasma glucose in the normal range; (2) if HbA1c goal was not reached, glipizide therapy was added; (3) if HbA1c goal was not reached by step 2, a morning dose of insulin was added and the oral agent was stopped; and (4) if HbA1c goal was not reached, multiple-dose insulin therapy was used. Results are shown in Figure 2. It is apparent from this study that the addition of an oral sulfonylurea agent to bedtime intermediate insulin achieved an acceptable HbA1c fall to 7.4%. However, to achieve the maximal drop in HbA1c (to 7.1%), it was necessary to more than double the dosage of insulin in the absence of oral agent administration.

Because sulfonylureas were available in the U.S. for many years before other agents were introduced, the greatest experience in published studies has been with the combination of insulin plus sulfonylurea. A meta-analysis of 16 studies reported an overall reduction in HbA1c of 1.1% and a decrease in bedtime NPH dosage of 12 U/day with this strategy compared with controls.[104] This approach has been termed BIDS (Bedtime Insulin, Day Time Sulfonylurea). It is apparent that a multitude of combinations of insulin and sulfonylureas can be created. For instance, one may use glargine insulin at bedtime or (70/30) or (75/25) insulin before supper in combination with a sulfonylurea. The key is to obtain and maintain a FBG in the case of 80–120 mg/dl.

Metformin and Bedtime Insulin

In type 2 diabetics who were poorly controlled on oral agents, Yki-Jarvinen et al. compared four different strategies, all of which had bedtime NPH as the initial step.[218] Results from this study (of 1 year duration) are summarized in Table 9.

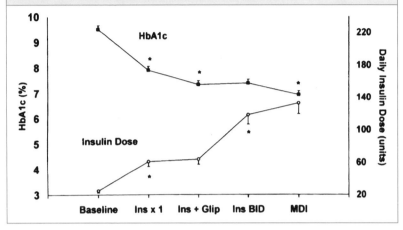

Figure 2. Comparison of HbA1c and insulin doses (mean ± SE) with treatment with evening insulin (Ins ×1), insulin + glipizide (Ins + Glip), twice-daily insulin (Ins BID) or multiple doses of insulin (MDI). The asterisks denote significant difference from the values in the preceding phase. (From Abraira C, et al. Diabetes Care 21:574–579, 1998, with permission.)

All combinations were effective in lowering HbA1c. Because the metformin plus bedtime NPH strategy was associated with less weight gain and an acceptable fall in HbA1c to a level of 7.2%, many physicians favor this approach as the first step in combination therapy with insulin and oral agents.

Other studies have supported the strategy of adding metformin therapy to insulin in type 2 diabetic patients with poorly controlled diabetes on insulin alone. In one randomized trial, metformin was increased gradually to top doses for 6 months and compared with placebo in 43 insulin-treated type 2 patients.[16] The metformin plus insulin group had a HbA1c fall of 2.5% compared with 1.6% in the placebo plus insulin group, despite a 29% increase in insulin dose in the second group. The

Table 9. Effects of Bedtime NPH and Daytime Oral Agents or Insulin in Type 2 Diabetes				
	Glyburide	Metformin	Gylbyuride + Metformin	AM NPH-Insulin
Number of patients	22	19	23	24
Change in HbA1c(%)	−1.9	−2.5	−2.1	−1.9
Increase in weight (lb)	8.6	2.0	7.9	10.1
Insulin dose (U)				
Bedtime	24	36	20	24
Morning				29

metformin group had a trend toward less weight gain (0.5 vs. 3.2 kg). A second study had similar results when metformin therapy was added to insulin in poorly controlled type 2 patients.[73]

Thiazolidinedione and Insulin

A promising approach to combination therapy is the addition of an insulin sensitizer (a thiazolidinedione) to insulin therapy. Because troglitazone was the first oral agent of this class approved for use in the U.S., most of the data from controlled studies deal with a combination of insulin and troglitazone. In one study, patients with type 2 diabetes were rendered euglycemic by insulin pump therapy before randomization to insulin pump therapy plus troglitazone vs. metformin.[220] Insulin requirements decreased 53% with troglitazone, and insulin sensitivity increased 29%. In the metformin plus insulin group, insulin requirements decreased 31%, and there was no increase in insulin sensitivity. These results are promising and now must be replicated in long-term studies with the newly approved agents pioglitazone and rosiglitazone, since troglitazone has been removed from the market. Preliminary short-term studies of the addition of pioglitazone or rosiglitazone to insulin in type 2 diabetes show a modest decrease in high insulin requirements and a fall of 1.0–1.2% in HbA1c when high doses of either agent are added to insulin in poorly controlled type 2 diabetic patients.[160,178] Long-term studies of this combination are under way.

Other Combinations of Oral Agents Plus Insulin

One promising approach is to target the postprandial glucose rise with rapid-acting insulin (lispro or aspart) before each meal, in combination with sulfonylurea therapy. In one study of patients who failed to reach HbA1c target on oral glyburide therapy, this strategy was associated with a greater fall in HbA1c at the end of 3 months (2.4%) than was seen in patients randomized to glyburide plus bedtime NPH (−1.8%).[23] This effect was seen despite of the fact that the overnight fasting blood glucose value was lower in the NPH plus glyburide group.

Insulin glargine has been approved by the FDA for use in the U.S. As discussed in the chapter on type 1 diabetes, this preparation gives a virtually peakless insulin profile in the majority of patients. When it is injected at bedtime, nocturnal hypoglycemia is less than with intermediate-acting insulins (NPH or lente),[129,161,175] and reproducibility of action appears to be better than with a single dose of ultralente insulin[129] (Fig. 3). Thus, insulin glargine may replace other insulins as the agent of choice to provide basal insulin coverage overnight in an attempt to produce FBG levels in the normal range. Furthermore, insulin glargine has a duration of action up to 24 hours, thus providing basal insulin to sup-

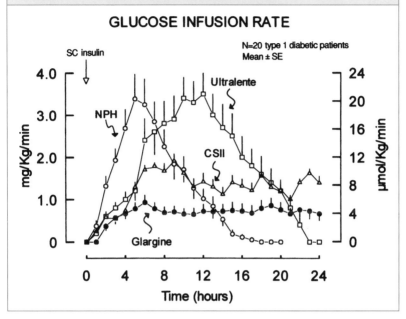

Figure 3. Rates of glucose infusion needed to maintain plasma glucose at a target value of 130 mg/dl after subcutaneous injection of four different insulin preparations. CSII = continuous subcutaneous lispro insulin infusion. (From Lepore M, et al. Diabetes 49:2142–2148, 2000, with permission.)

plement the daytime oral agent or insulin plan. Long-term studies with this new insulin in combination with oral agents are under way, and the results are eagerly awaited.

Benefits of Bedtime Insulin

Metabolic benefits from the use of insulin at bedtime include the following:

- Provides basal insulin action to achieve normal fasting blood glucose and to help achieve normal postprandial blood glucose values.
- Suppresses the increased overnight hepatic glucose production, which causes fasting hyperglycemia in uncontrolled diabetes.
- Suppresses plasma free fatty acid levels, improves lipoprotein metabolism, suppresses hepatic glucose production, and helps overcome insulin resistance.
- Counteracts the increase in insulin resistance before awakening (the dawn phenomenon).

Patient acceptance of this regimen is generally good. By targeting FBG, one key measurement is all that is needed when bedtime insulin is started. Compliance is usually improved with one vs. two or three daily insulin injections, and the system of insulin adjustment is easily understood by most patients. With long-term use, weight gain may be less than with multiple insulin injection strategies. Finally, the development of new oral agents and insulins may lead to improved overall glycemic control and the prevention of progression of microvascular complications.

A Practical Approach to Patients with Elevated HbA1c While on Two Oral Agent(s)

- Continue two oral agents.
- Add single bedtime dose of NPH, lente, or glargine insulin.
- Alternatively, add equal doses of ultralente before breakfast and supper as the basal dose.
- Choose dosage empirically. Because obese type 2 patients who have failed control on oral agents generally need ≥ 1 U/kg as total insulin replacement, a safe initial bedtime dose of basal insulin is 0.2–0.3 U/kg. For nonobese patients, use 0.1–0.2 U/kg.
- Instruct the patient to do daily FBG determinations.
- Ask patient to adjust bedtime dose weekly, with a goal of attaining consistent FPG values of 80–120 mg/dl. Usually, weekly increments of about 10–30% of the original bedtime dose are safe and increase effectiveness of glycemic control.
- Instruct the patient to send the FBG and insulin dosage decisions by fax, e-mail, or telephone every 2 weeks for feedback. Ask the patient to call if hypoglycemia occurs.
- Begin monitoring of daytime premeal (and periodic 2-hour postprandial) blood glucose levels after target FBG of 80–120 mg/dl is met. Final bedtime dose is often 0.4–0.5 U/kg.
- Start 70/30 or 75/25 insulin before breakfast if HbA1c goals are not met after 3–6 months on maximal doses of both oral agents and bedtime insulin

Multiple-dose Insulin Therapy

As noted in the natural history of type 2 diabetes (Fig. 2, Chapter 8), there is usually a need for a progressive increase in antidiabetic therapy to achieve the recommended HbA1c goals. Unfortunately, because long-term collaborative trials have not yet achieved the rather stringent HbA1c goal of < 7% in the majority of patients with type 2 diabetes, it is necessary to make empirical recommendations. Patients who may be in need of a multiple-dose insulin regimen are usually overweight type 2 diabetics with known diabetes of 10–15 years or longer. Generally, such patients have failed metabolic control with single or multiple oral agents and have progressed to the stage of bedtime intermediate or long-acting insulin along with daytime administration of one or more oral agents. Further action in indicated if HbA1c is > 8%, and the goal is to achieve a HbA1c level of < 7% without undue weight gain or frequent episodes of hypoglycemia. Although a target HbA1c of ≤ 6.5% has been recommended by one group, the benefit-to-risk ratio of this approach has not been clearly demonstrated.

Split-Mixed Insulin Twice Daily

One approach was carefully studied in obese type 2 diabetic patients.[91] NPH plus regular Insulin was given twice daily, before breakfast and supper, and doses were adjusted biweekly to achieve excellent diabetic control. This goal was achieved using a total insulin dosage of about 1 U/kg, with an NPH: regular ratio of 75:25. Approximately 50% of the insulin was given before breakfast and 50% before supper. There was a decrease in hepatic glucose output of 44% and an increase in insulin sensitivity of 17% over the 6 months of the study. Hypoglycemia was rare, but there was a weight gain of about 8.7kg. This study illustrates several critical points in insulin management of obese type 2 diabetics:

- Large insulin doses (≥1 U/kg) are needed.
- Split-mixed insulin in a 70/30 or 75/25 ratio of intermediate- to rapid-acting insulin, divided equally before breakfast and supper is safe and effective.
- Severe hypoglycemia is rarely seen.
- Metabolic improvement is illustrated by a modest increase in insulin sensitivity and a major decrease in hepatic glucose output.
- Weight gain is the most troubling side effect.

Thus, one may initiate split-mixed insulin therapy in obese type 2 diabetics in a regimen comparable to that used in this study. It is prudent to start with a total daily dose of 0.5–0.6 U/kg of 70/30 or 75/25 insulin, split evenly before breakfast and supper. Adjust dosages upward every week or two until premeal normal blood glucose values are achieved.

Alternative Approaches

There are many alternative approaches to insulin therapy in type 2 diabetes. Many physicians prefer to use intermediate insulin or insulin glargine at bedtime to control the FBG and to administer 70/30 or 70/25 insulin before breakfast as the second dose. There are no direct comparisons of this method with the split-mixed insulin twice-daily approach.

With the availability of the new rapid-acting insulin analogues, lispro and aspart, physicians now have the opportunity to ask patients to use one of these insulins immediately before each meal and then to add a bedtime dosage of glargine or an intermediate insulin to control FBG. An obvious disadvantage is the need for four daily injections, but if inhaled rapid-acting insulin[33,146,186] is approved, it could replace the premeal injections.

Another popular strategy is to use ultralente insulin as about 60% of the total dose. Divide this into equal doses before breakfast and supper, and mix immediately before injection with rapid-acting insulin to cover the meals. Prescribe a third dose of rapid-acting insulin at lunchtime.

What is the Best Approach?

There is no evidence-based answer to this question. Currently, many trials of different combinations of insulin and oral agents are under way. Until the results of these trials are known, here is an arbitrary overview of an approach to achieving excellent glycemic control in obese type 2 patients who have failed on single- or dual-oral agent therapy:

1. Instruct the patient again about the importance of a caloric-restricted nutrition plan along with an exercise conditioning program in anticipation of weight gain.
2. Try a combination of an oral insulin sensitizer plus a stimulator of insulin secretion as the daytime regimen. Use metformin as the initial agent in overweight patients.
3. Use a split-mix insulin preparation before supper or insulin glargine at bedtime to achieve FBG levels in the normal range. Alternative insulins are ultralente before supper or NPH/lente at bedtime.
   - If target HbA1c goals (ideally, <7% without hypoglycemia) are not met, add a morning dose of split-mix insulin before breakfast.
   - If target HbA1c goals are still not met, drop the oral agents and push the two doses of insulin to the necessary high doses (usually ≥ 1 U/kg).
   - Try different strategies until something works!

Glucagon-like Peptide

Glucagon-like peptide-1 (GLP-1) has been shown to stimulate insulin secretion. In one study, GLP-1 was infused at a constant rate subcutaneously for 6 weeks in a group of 10 patients with type 2 diabetes.[222] There was a significant decrease in plasma glucose and a fall in HbA1c of 1.35%. Pancreatic beta-cell function improved, as did insulin sensitivity. Free fatty acid levels fell, and gastric emptying was inhibited. Appetite was reduced, and body weight decreased by 1.9 kg. Because GLP-1 has a rapid half-life, research has focused on preparations that would extend its duration of action. One compound, exendin-4, a peptide isolated from the oral secretions of the gila monster, has such activity. In humans, synthetic exendin-4 delays gastric emptying, suppresses appetite, and contributes to weight loss. Postprandial plasma glucose and triglyceride levels are decreased. Animal studies have shown that exendin-4 stimulates differentiation of pancreatic beta cells from progenitor cells and beta cell proliferation in rats.

This combination of beta-cell stimulation, appetite suppression, and weight reduction makes GLP-1 a promising agent for potential application to the therapy of people with type 2 diabetes. Long-term studies of efficacy and safety are needed, and research will continue in an attempt to develop orally active compounds that utilize the GLP-1 system.

Key Points: Insulin Therapy in Type 2 Diabetes

- Insulin therapy, alone or in combination with one or two oral agents, is usually needed in type 2 diabetic patients with diabetes duration of over 10 years.
- Combination therapy of an oral agent (or two) during the day and evening or bedtime insulin is often an effective strategy. Insulin glargine at bedtime is an excellent choice to avoid nocturnal hypoglycemia.
- Some evidence favors bedtime NPH plus daytime metformin as the first step in combination therapy.
- Addition of an insulin stimulator to the above regimen is often the next step.
- An alternative strategy is to add a thiazolidinedione.
- If these steps fail, add a morning dosage of split-mixed insulin before breakfast.
- Total insulin dosage in obese type 2 patients usually is ≥ 1 U/kg if insulin is used alone.
- Intensive glycemic control with insulin in type 2 diabetic patients decreases hepatic glucose output and increases insulin sensitivity.
- Weight gain is a component of successful regimens of intensive glycemic control in type 2 diabetes unless nutrition planning with caloric restriction and an exercise program are successfully implemented.
- There is no evidence-based answer for which of many possible regimens to prescribe. Physicians currently favor a combination of insulin plus one or two oral agents to avoid the use of very high insulin doses.

Hypertension

Rationale for Intensive Blood Pressure Management in Type 2 Diabetes

Hypertension is a prevalent and important problem in type 2 diabetes. Its prevalence in type 2 diabetes is approximately double that in nondiabetic controls. At least 40% of Caucasian patients with type 2 diabetes have blood pressures $\geq$ 140/90 mmHg by age 50, and 60% have hypertension by age 70. Prevalence is highest in African Americans, Hispanics and American Indians. In a survey of 1507 adults with diabetes (NHANES III), 71% were found to have high blood pressure, defined as $\geq$ 130/85 mmHg or on antihypertensive medication.[71] Only 57% were being treated, and 29% were unaware that they had hypertension. Only 12% had BP < 130/85 mmHg, and 45% had a BP < 140/90 mmHg. With the current goals of therapy set at achieving a blood pressure $\leq$ 130/80 mmHg, it is apparent that the vast majority of people with type 2 diabetes in the U.S. require therapy for blood pressure elevation and that present efforts at control are inadequate.

Epidemiologic evidence makes clear that elevated blood pressure contributes to stroke, microalbuminuria, renal failure, cardiovascular death, peripheral vascular disease, and retinopathy progression in people with type 2 diabetes.[13,14,21,58,72,188] These epidemiologic associations imply strongly that reduction of blood pressure would have a number of beneficial effects if practiced effectively in type 2 diabetes. Fortunately, we now have solid information from a number of prospective controlled trials that such therapy is highly effective. Furthermore, these trials have given insight into the levels of systolic and diastolic blood pressure that are associated with increasing risks and the optimal blood pressure goals to achieve with antihypertensive agents.

Many epidemiologic studies have demonstrated that systolic and diastolic blood pressures have a strong and continuously positive association with cardiovascular events. Recently, Vasan et al. reported the impact of various degrees of blood pressure elevation on the risk of cardiovascular events in a 10-year follow-up of the Framingham cohort.[209] On the basis of criteria from the Joint National Committee on Prevention, Detection, Evaluation, and Treatment of High Blood Pressure (JNC VI) and the World Health Organization and the International Society of Hypertension (WHO-ISH), they recognized three classifications: (1) optimal (systolic pressure < 120 mmHg and diastolic pressure < 80 mmHg; (2) normal (systolic pressure 120–129 mmHg or diastolic pressure 80–84 mmHg); (3) high normal (systolic pressure 130–139 mmHg or diastolic pressure 85–89 mmHg). These classifications allowed analysis of the effects of a series of blood pressures below the older guidelines for hypertension of $\leq$ 140/90 mmHg. They found that, compared with normal blood pressure, high normal BP was associated with a cardiovascular risk factor-adjusted ratio of 2.5 in women and 16.2 in men. Although this population was primarily made up of nondiabetic people, it is likely that even greater risks would be found in type 2 diabetic subjects.

In any case, there is a clear rationale for aggressive blood pressure treatment in people with type 2 diabetes.[14] Current recommendations have evolved from impressive results from a number of intervention trials. Key trials have provided evidence that blood pressure-lowering is an extremely important form of preventive therapy for cardiovascular events in people with type 2 diabetes.

The first of these trials was an examination of calcium channel blocker therapy for hypertension in type 2 diabetics with isolated systolic hypertension. The analysis was done in 492 diabetic subjects and 4203 nondiabetic subjects who were enrolled in the Isolated Systolic Hypertension in Europe (Syst-Eur) trial.[200] The subjects were all ≥ 60 years of age and had systolic blood pressures ≥ 160 mmHg, and diastolic BP < 95 mmHg. They were randomized to the calcium channel blocker nitrendipine (10–40 mg/day) with possible addition or substitution of the ACE inhibitor enalapril (5–20 mg/day), hydrochlorothiazide (12.5–25mg/day), or both vs. placebo. The active drugs were adjusted to reduce systolic BP by at least 20 mmHg and to less than 150 mmHg. Results are shown in Table 10. In the diabetic subjects, there was a highly significant reduction in total mortality (41%), cardiovascular mortality (70%), cardiovascular events (62%), and fatal and nonfatal strokes (69%). These effects were significantly greater in the diabetic patients than in the nondiabetic groups. Thus, antihypertensive treatment of diabetic subjects with systolic hypertension, beginning with calcium channel blockade, was particularly beneficial compared with nondiabetic subjects. This study confirmed and extended results from the Systolic Hypertension in the Elderly Program,[48] in which diuretic-based antihypertensive therapy in non–insulin-treated people with type 2 diabetes was associated with a significant 34% reduction in the risk for major cardiovascular events. The mean blood pressure reduction was only 7/2 mmHg from a mean baseline BP of 170/77 mmHg.

Another major trial to show the benefits of blood pressure reduction in people with type 2 diabetes is the UKPDS tight blood pressure trial.[202,204,206] This large substudy was embedded in the main trial, which explored the effects of a policy of intensive glycemic regulation vs. one of less stringent blood glucose control. In the hypertension trial, 1148 type 2 diabetic patients with untreated hypertension (systolic BP ≥ 160 and/or diastolic BP ≥ 90 mmHg) or on therapy for hypertension (BP ≥ 150/85 mmHg) were randomly assigned to tight BP control vs. less tight control. In the tight control group, the goal BP was < 150/85 mmHg, and patients were randomized into treatment with an ACE inhibitor (captopril) or a beta blocker (atenolol) as original therapy. If BP goals were not met by maximal doses, additional drugs were added: furosemide, nifedipine, methyldopa, and/or prazosin. In the less tight control group, BP was < 180/105 mmHg, and therapy with ACE inhibitors or beta blockers was avoided. Results are shown in Table 10.

	No. DM	Mean No.	Baseline BP	Drop in	Reduction[†] In:		
Trial	Patients	of Years	(mmHg)	BP (mmHg)	CV Mort	CV Events	Strokes
Syst-Eur	492	2	178/84	8.6/3.9	70%	62%	69%
UKPDS	1148	8.4	159/94	10/5	32%	21%	44%
HOT	1501	3.8	170/105	20–24/26–30	67%*	30%*	30%*

Table 10. Effects of Blood Pressure Reduction on Cardiovascular Events in Hypertensive Type 2 Diabetics

*Comparison is between group randomized to diastolic BP ≤ 90 mmHg vs. ≤ 80 mmHg
[†]All risk reductions significant except CV events in UKPDS.
References to studies are included in the text.

There was a 32% reduction in the risk of cardiovascular death and a 44% reduction in the risk of stroke. Retinopathy risk was also assessed, and a 37% reduction was seen, primarily in the risk for photocoagulation. Results in the group randomized first to ACE inhibitor therapy were the same as those initially assigned to atenolol treatment. To achieve BP goals, the majority of patients in the tight control group required two or more drugs. By the end of 9 years, 29% of those assigned to tight blood pressure control required three or more drugs.

Another major trial of intensive blood pressure lowering was the Hypertension Optimal Treatment (HOT) randomized trial,[87,88] a large study that enrolled 18,790 patients with hypertension and diastolic BP between 100 and 118 mmHg. They were randomly assigned to a diastolic BP target of ≤ 90, ≤ 85, or ≤ 80 mmHg. The calcium channel blocker felodipine (5mg) was given as baseline therapy, and other agents were added in a five-step protocol. ACE inhibitors or beta blockers were added at step 2, dosage titration of felodipine at step 3, titration of ACE inhibitor or beta blocker at step 4, and addition of a diuretic at step 5.

There were 1501 patients with diabetes mellitus in the study. Because the age range was 50–80 years, the majority of these patients had type 2 diabetes. In the group randomized to ≤ 80 mmHg, the risk of major cardiovascular events was halved in comparison with the ≤ 90 mmHg group. The achieved BP's were 81.1 and 85.2 mmHg, respectively. Cardiovascular mortality and stroke were also significantly lower in the ≤ 80 mmHg, vs. ≤ 90 mmHg group (Table 10).

Support for achieving a diastolic BP ≤ 80 mmHg has been provided by the Appropriate Blood Pressure Control in Diabetes (ABCD) Trial.[183] In this study of 480 type 2 diabetic subjects with baseline diastolic BP of 80–90 mmHg, randomization to a strategy to lower diastolic BP by 10 mmHg with either enalapril or nisoldipine resulted in a slowing of progression to incipient and overt diabetic nephropathy, a decrease in progression of diabetic retinopathy, and a diminution in the incidence of stroke.

Thus, solid evidence favors the guidelines to lower blood pressure to ≤ 130/80 mmHg in type 2 diabetic subjects.

Management of Elevated Blood Pressure

Collectively, these studies argue convincingly for a policy of intensive blood pressure lowering in people with type 2 diabetes. Significant and impressive reductions in the risks of cardiovascular mortality, cardiovascular events, and stroke were generally seen and were consistently greater in the diabetic than in the nondiabetic groups. Furthermore, a decrease in progression of renal disease and retinopathy occurred in the ABCD trial. Although earlier studies had suggested increased cardiovascular risk associated with calcium channel therapy (dihydropiridine class), this finding was not confirmed in the Syst-Eur, HOT, or ABCD Trial. In a recent review of five studies, Bakris et al. found that an average of 3.2 antihypertensive agents were needed to achieve more stringent blood pressure control.[21] In these trials, the major endpoints evaluated were cardiovascular events. Other trials, to be discussed in another section, presented strong support for ACE inhibitor or angiotensin II receptor blocker therapy to slow progression of diabetic renal disease. Furthermore, the UKPDS showed a beneficial effect of tight blood pressure control on progression of retinopathy to laser therapy despite a rise in HbA1c to 8.3%. In the ABCD Trial, HbA1c was in the 10–11.5% range. The UKPDS also showed that tight control of blood pressure substantially reduced the cost of complications and had a cost-effectiveness ratio that compared favorably with accepted health care programs.[202] Finally, as discussed in another section, ACE inhibitor therapy has now been shown to significantly lower cardiovascular risk with minimal BP change in diabetic patients who are at high risk for such events.

Recommendations for antihypertensive therapy in people with type 2 diabetes are given in Table 11. Many physicians use the strategy followed in the HOT Trial: start with a low dose of the first agent, add low

Table 11. One Method of Choosing Antihypertensive Agents in People with Type 2 Diabetes
1. Start therapy: BP ≥ 130/80 mmHg.
2. Goal of therapy: BP ≤ 120/70 mmHg.
3. Restrict dietary sodium to < 2500 mg/day.
4. First agent: low-dose ACE inhibitor (or ARB).
5. Second agent: low-dose thiazide (loop diuretic if serum creatinine ≥ 1.8 mg/dl).
6. Third agent: low-dose calcium channel blocker.
7. Fourth agent: low-dose beta blocker (if pulse rate > 70 beats/min).
8. Titrate doses upward (in sequence) to achieve goal BP.
9. Add other agents if necessary (alpha blockers, vasodilators).

doses of additional agents, then titrate to higher doses if goals are not reached. In any case, recognize that two to four antihypertensive agents are often necessary.

Key Points: Intensive Management of Hypertension in Type 2 Diabetes

- ⊙ Elevated blood pressure in type 2 diabetes contributes to retinopathy, microalbuminuria, renal failure, cardiovascular deaths, strokes, and peripheral vascular disease.
- ⊙ At least 40% of Caucasians with type 2 diabetes have hypertension by age 50 and 60% by age 70. Overall, 71% of adults with diabetes have hypertension (BP ≥ 130/85 mmHg).
- ⊙ Prevalence is highest in African and Hispanic Americans and American Indians.
- ⊙ Both systolic and diastolic blood pressure have a strong, continuous relationship with cardiovascular events in longitudinal studies.
- ⊙ Epidemiologic data from the Framingham Study indicate that 120/80 mmHg is an optimal blood pressure.
- ⊙ Consistent evidence from controlled clinical trials indicates that reduction of elevated systolic and/or diastolic blood pressures in people with type 2 diabetes leads to major reduction in cardiovascular risks.
- ⊙ Therapy should be started at BP ≥ 130/80 mmHg with a goal of ≤ 120/70 mmHg in type 2 diabetes. Thus, treatment of blood pressure should be instituted in the majority of people with type 2 diabetes.
- ⊙ A recommended strategy is to start with low dose of ACE inhibitor or angiotensin receptor blocker. Add low doses of a thiazide, calcium channel blocker, and beta blocker. If target BP of 120/70 mmHg is not reached, raise doses consecutively. Add an alpha blocker, vasodilators, and other agents if necessary.
- ⊙ Most patients with hypertension and type 2 diabetes require two or more agents to achieve recommended BP goals.

Nephropathy

Rationale for Intensive Management of Nephropathy in Type 2 Diabetes.

An earlier chapter indicated that the incidence of end-stage renal disease in the U.S. is rising and that over 50% of patients started on dialysis are now found to have diabetes. Because type 2 diabetes is such a prevalent disease, the majority of new cases of ESRD are patients with type 2 diabetes. Epidemiologic data indicate that hyperglycemia and hypertension are major risk factors, and excellent evidence from collaborative trials indicates that intensive glycemic control slows progression of incipient nephropathy (microalbuminuria) to overt nephropathy (24-hour urinary albumin > 300 mg). It is also clear that effective blood pressure control delays or prevents progression to ESRD.

Tabaei et al. questioned whether microalbuminuria is a sensitive and specific indicator of diabetic nephropathy.[193] This issue was explored by Parving et al., who reviewed results from 16 studies and concluded that microalbuminuria is the best documented predictor of diabetic nephropathy in both type 1 and type 2 diabetes.[155] The mean rate of patients developing nephropathy after 2–4 years of type 1 diabetes in seven studies was approximately 7.5%/year (range: 5.5–13%). In nine studies, the mean rate after up to 9 years of type 2 diabetes was about 6%/year (range: 2.4–9.3%). Accordingly, yearly measurement of urinary microalbumin in people with type 1 and type 2 diabetes is an ADA standard of care.[10,13]

Inhibition of the action of the renin-angiotensin system appears to have an independent renoprotective effect. Hypertension, high protein intake, smoking, hypercholesterolemia, and insulin resistance have been identified as possible contributors to diabetic nephropathy. Although collaborative trial evidence is either negative or unavailable, most physicians include attention to these risk markers in the comprehensive approach to intensive management of nephropathy. People with type 2 diabetes and hypertension have not only a high incidence of renal insufficiency but also a high prevalence of a constellation of other cardiovascular risk factors, including microalbuminuria, dyslipidemia, prothrombotic state, and left ventricular hypertrophy. Thus, a multifactorial approach to the treatment of the type 2 diabetic patient with renal disease is clearly supported by correlative analyses and positive collaborative trial evidence.[10,69] However, despite increased awareness and modification of guidelines for care of people with type 2 diabetes, the incidence of reported therapy for ESRD in diabetes has had a linear rise since 1982.[21]

One factor that may be of importance in this increase is a slight decline in cardiovascular mortality in diabetes, leading to more patients who survive until reaching ESRD. However, as previously discussed, cardiovascular mortality in the past 10–20 years declined minimally among men with diabetes and actually rose among women with diabetes in follow-up examinations of NHANES-1 cohorts[79,80] It is more likely that a failure to achieve recommended goals for glycemia, blood pressure, and other risk factors in the past two decades in people with type 2 diabetes is the major contributor to this phenomenon. Translation of study results that recommend inhibition of the renin-angiotensin system to the general practice of medicine is just beginning. In addition, there has been an increasing incidence in type 2 diabetes in the U.S., as well as increasing numbers of type 2 patients in the ethnic groups with a high incidence of ESRD. The good news is that recent prospective, randomized trial data give good evidence that progression to ESRD can be delayed or prevented by aggressive multifactorial therapy in type 2 as well as type 1 diabetes.

Management of Nephropathy

A variety of renal disease markers and endpoints were studied in the tight blood pressure control trial of the UKPDS.[204,206] Hypertensive subjects with type 2 diabetes (who were enrolled in the parent trial of glucose control) were randomly assigned to tight control of blood pressure (goal < 150/85 mmHg) or less tight control (goal < 180/105 mmHg). By 6 years of study, a smaller proportion of patients in the tight control group had urinary albumin excretion ≥ 50 mg/L—a 29% reduction in risk (p = 0.009). There was a trend toward reduction in albuminuria ≥ 300 mg/L of 39%, but it did not quite reach statistical significance (p = 0.061). The numbers of patients who had renal failure (or death from renal failure) also tended to be less in the intensively managed group, but the numbers were small and not significantly different from the other group.

In another comparative study, beta blockers and ACE inhibitors were equally effective strategies in reducing declining kidney function in hypertensive type 2 patients with nephropathy.[148] There has been great interest in the effects of ACE inhibitors and/or angiotensin receptor blockers (ARBs) on renal disease in people with type 2 diabetes. In an early study, Ravid et al showed a long-term renoprotective effect of ACE inhibitor therapy in type 2 diabetes.[162] This study was influenced by earlier studies by Brenner's group[28] on the beneficial effects of ACE inhibitor therapy on intraglomerular hypertension in diabetic animals and by positive results from studies by Lewis et al. of ACE inhibitor therapy in type 1 diabetes.[131] Recent retrospective analyses of ACE inhibitor trials indicated that ACE inhibitors should provide long-term beneficial effects, even in patients with an initial rise in serum creatinine.[182] Renoprotective effects of ACE inhibitor therapy have been noted in early diabetic nephropathy, even in patients with normal blood pressure.[183]

The beneficial effects of ACE inhibitor therapy may not be due solely to blood pressure-lowering. In the MICRO-HOPE Substudy of the HOPE trial, 3577 people with diabetes, aged 55 or older, were randomly assigned to ramipril (10 mg/day) or placebo therapy.[90,196,197] These high-risk diabetic patients had a history of cardiovascular disease or at least one cardiovascular risk factor (cholesterol > 200 mg/dl, HDL cholesterol < 40 mg/dl, hypertension, microalbuminuria, or current smoking). The 24% reduction in progression to overt nephropathy (24-hour urinary albumin > 300 mg) reached statistical significance (p = 0.027). The effect was independent of blood pressure reduction and may have been due to the lowering of intraglomerular capillary pressure.

Collaborative trial data on the use of ARBs in type 2 diabetic patients have now appeared. Earlier studies suggested that ARBs could lower urinary protein excretion and that the effect was independent of their antihypertensive action. Three large multicenter clinical trials in hypertensive type 2 diabetic patients with nephropathy suggest that ARBs may be as effective as ACE inhibitors in blood pressure reduction and renoprotection.[29,96,130,156] Because ARBs do not increase bradykinin levels, they are not associated with cough, an occasional side effect of ACE inhibitor therapy. Evidence indicates that angiotensin II may be produced from sites independent of the angiotensin I to II pathway, suggesting that ARBs may be valuable as ancillary drugs to ACE inhibitor therapy in selected patients. In two studies, dual blockade of the renin-angiotensin system was more effective than single blockade in patients with type 2 diabetes, hypertension and microalbuminuria.[141,177]

Prospective trial evidence indicates that a multifactorial approach is successful in slowing progression to nephropathy (albumin excretion > 300 mg/24 hr) in people with type 2 diabetes and microalbuminuria. In the 4-year Steno Type 2 Randomized Study, 160 patients with type 2 diabetes and microalbuminuria were randomized to standard or intensive treatment.[69] Intensive treatment was stepwise implementation of behavior modification and intensive therapy targeting hyperglycemia, hypertension, dyslipidemia, and microalbuminuria. The intensively treated group had significant reductions in HbA1c, improved lipid profiles, and a fall in blood pressure, all of which were greater than in the standard therapy group. Progression to the primary endpoint of nephropathy was decreased by 73%.

Finally, one analysis concluded that treating all patients with type 2 diabetes with ACE inhibitors is cost-effective compared with screening for microalbuminuria or gross proteinuria.[75] This interesting approach requires further study; at this stage, it has not been adopted as a standard of care by the ADA.

Key Points: Intensive Management of Nephropathy

- There has been a linear increase in the incidence of ESRD in the U.S. since 1982.
- Intensive glycemic control slows progression from microalbuminuria to clinical nephropathy (albumin exretion > 300 mg/24 hr).

Key Points (*Continued*)

• Strong clinical trial evidence indicates that both systolic and diastolic blood pressure should be aggressively treated in type 2 diabetes.

• A standard of care is to check for microalbuminuria annually in type 2 diabetes, starting at time of diagnosis or earlier (i.e., in patients with metabolic syndrome).

• The first indicator of renal damage is microalbuminuria (30–300 mg albumin/24 hours or 30 μg/mg creatinine in a spot urine specimen).

• ACE inhibitor therapy delays or prevents progression from microalbuminuria to nephropathy (> 300 mg albumin/24-hr urine).

• Treatment for hypertension in type 2 diabetes has a goal BP < 130/80 mmHg. (i.e. 120/70 mmHg)

• ACE inhibitors and ARBs lower urinary protein excretion and prevent progression of renal insufficiency in type 2 diabetes.

• The beneficial effects of ACE inhibitor therapy on diabetic nephropathy are not explained entirely by reduction in systemic blood pressure.

• The beneficial effects of ACE inhibitor therapy may be due to reduction of intraglomerular capillary pressure as well as systemic blood pressure.

• A multifactorial approach to the treatment of blood pressure, glycemia, lipids, and microalbuminuria has been shown to decrease progression to nephropathy in type 2 diabetes by 73%.

Lipids/Lipoproteins

A Consensus for Intensive Management of Lipids and Lipoproteins in Type 2 Diabetes

Type 2 diabetes has long been known to be associated with accelerated coronary heart disease.[1, 188] Typically, people with type 2 diabetes have an atherogenic lipid profile, characterized by elevated plasma triglycerides, low plasma HDL cholesterol levels, and increased population of small, dense LDL particles. An important consideration is that these alterations are frequently seen in the very early stages of type 2 diabetes, during the stage of impaired glucose tolerance or metabolic syndrome. Thus, even before the appearance of fasting hyperglycemia and a definitive diagnosis of diabetes, patients are at high risk for cardiovascular events due, at least in part, to persistent dyslipidemia.[150] Fortunately, clinical trial evidence has rapidly accumulated to support aggressive lipid-lowering treatment strategies in type 2 diabetes.

The ADA[12] and the National Cholesterol Education Program (NCEP) Adult Treatment Panel III (ATP III)[60] have now joined forces in recommending that diabetic patients be treated for lipid alterations with the same intensity as nondiabetics with established coronary heart disease. This is a major policy shift for NCEP(ATP III). In its recent report, this group recognized that people with diabetes or metabolic syndrome have extremely high cardiovascular risks.[60] The new features of this important report are as follows:

1. Focus on multiple risk factors
   - Raises persons with diabetes without CHD, most of whom display multiple risk factors, to the risk level of CHD risk equivalent.
   - Uses Framingham projections of 10-year absolute CHD risk (i.e., the percent probability of having a CHD event in 10 years) to identify certain patients with multiple (2+) risk factors for more intensive treatment.
   - Identifies persons with multiple metabolic risk factors (metabolic syndrome) as candidates for intensified therapeutic lifestyle changes.

2. Modifications of lipid and lipoprotein classification
   - Identifies LDL cholesterol <100 mg/dl as optimal.
   - Raises categorical low HDL cholesterol from < 35mg/dl to < 40 mg/dL (men) because the latter value is a better measure of depressed HDL.
   - Lowers the triglyceride classification cutpoints to give more attention to moderate elevations (>150 mg/dl).

3. Support for implementation
   - Recommends a complete lipoprotein profile every 5 years in patients ≥ 20 years of age. Fasting levels of total cholesterol, LDL cholesterol, HDL cholesterol, and triglycerides as the preferred initial test.
   - Encourages use of plant stanols/sterols and viscous (soluble) fiber as therapeutic dietary options to enhance lowering of LDL cholesterol.
   - Presents strategies for promoting adherence to therapeutic lifestyle changes and drug therapies.
   - Recommends treatment beyond LDL-lowering for persons with triglycerides ≥ 200 mg/dl.

The recommendations in this report have been eagerly awaited by the diabetes community for many years. In the first report of the National Cholesterol Education Program[164] the emphasis was on lowering of LDL cholesterol as a primary prevention strategy in people with high LDL cholesterol levels (> 160 mg/dl) or with levels of 130–159 mg/dl plus at least two coronary risk factors. Diabetes was viewed as a coronary risk factor and received minimal rating in the Framingham risk score. Yet the major cause of death in type 2 diabetes was clearly cardiovascular disease, and it was known that cardiovascular risk was well in excess of the risk in non-diabetics. The report did not recognize this issue. Simultaneously, Gerald Reaven demonstrated in his Banting Lecture at the ADA in 1988, that "syndrome X" was associated with a high cardiovascular risk.[163] This observation catalyzed intense interest in this entity among diabetes specialists.

ATP II focused on patients with established coronary artery disease and recommended intensive LDL cholesterol (LDL-C) lowering to ≤ 100 mg/dl. Diabetes was not viewed as a separate high-risk issue. Meanwhile, evidence continued to mount indicating that most people with type 2 diabetes had an extraordinarily high-risk for coronary artery events.[3,79,80,109,188] Finally, it was conclusively demonstrated that the risk for the first heart attack in type 2 diabetes equaled that in nondiabetics who had already had a myocardial infarction.[84] Furthermore, although promising reductions in the risk for cardiovascular events were seen in the general population over the past 2–3 decades, little benefit was seen in men with diabetes, and the cardiovascular event rates actually increased in women with diabetes over the same period.[79]

The ATP III Report gives an evidenced-based approach that focuses first on LDL-C as the primary target of therapy.[60,123] The major change in approach is the recognition that diabetes is a coronary heart disease (CHD) equivalent rather than merely a cardiovascular risk factor. Thus, people with diabetes are to be treated as if they had CHD, and aggressive lowering of LDL-C to 100 mg/dl or below is the goal. This guideline accord with earlier recommendations made by the ADA and removes any confusion that may have existed in the past.

The ADA approaches lipid therapy in adults with diabetes by defining levels of cardiovascular risk (Table 12).[12] The ADA then defines the LDL-C goal as ≤ 100 mg/dl, which is to be achieved by exercise, medical nutrition, and pharmacologic therapy (if needed) in patients with or without cardiovascular disease.

A specific recommendation for patients with metabolic syndrome or diabetes who have LDL-C levels > 130 mg/dl is to initiate drug therapy (i.e., statins) if therapeutic lifestyle changes (TLC) cannot achieve an LDL-C goal of < 100 mg/dl. In the case of intermediate LDL-C levels of

Table 12. Risk Assessment Based on Lipoprotein Levels in Adults with Diabetes			
Risk Level	LDL-C	HDL-C*	Triglycerides
High	≥ 130	< 35	≥400 mg/dl
Borderline	100–129	35–45	200–399 mg/dl
Low	< 100	> 45	<200 mg/dl

LDL-C = low density lipoprotein cholesterol; HDL-C = high-density lipoprotein cholesterol.
*Values in women should be increased by 10 mg/dl.

100–129 mg/dl, both the ADA and the NCEP (ATP III) make similar TLC recommendations. However, if this approach fails, the ADA favors pharmacologic treatment with a statin, and the NCEP (ATP III) group gives the option of statin therapy or drugs that primarily modify triglycerides and HDL-C (nicotinic acid or fibrates). Clinical judgment must be used for patients in this category.

Total Lifestyle Changes

The recommendations for TLC changes also are now similar from the two groups. The essential features of TLC, as defined by NCEP (ATIII), are as follows:

- Reduced intakes of saturated fats (< 7% of total calories) and cholesterol (< 200 mg/day)
- Therapeutic options for enhancing LDL-lowering, such as plant stanols/sterols (2 gm/day) and increased viscous (soluble) fiber (10–25 gm/day)
- Weight reduction
- Increased physical activity

The nutrient composition of the TLC diet is shown in Table 13. This diet differs only slightly from the nutrition plan recommended by the ADA. In particular, total fat may range from 25% to 35%, particularly if saturated fats and trans fatty acids are kept very low. The ADA recommends that fat intake be < 30% but acknowledges that monounsaturated fat may be substituted for carbohydrates. The focus is on patients with high plasma triglyceride and low HDL-C levels, a problem which has been recognized for over 25 years in type 2 diabetes.[133]

Table 13. Nutrient Composition of the TLC Diet	
Nutrient	**Recommended Intake**
Saturated fat*	Less than 7% of total calories
Polyunsaturated fat	Up to 10% of total calories
Monounsaturated fat	Up to 20% of total calories
Total fat	25–35% of total calories
Carbohydrate†	50–60% of total calories
Fiber	20–30 grams per day
Protein	Approximately 15% of total calories
Cholesterol	Less than 200 mg/day
Total calories (energy)‡	Balance energy intake and expenditure to maintain desirable body weight/prevent weight gain

*Trans fatty acids are another LDL-raising fat that should be kept at a low intake.
†Carbohydrate should be derived predominantly from foods rich in complex carbohydrates including grains, especially whole grains, fruits, and vegetables.
‡Daily energy expenditure should include at least moderate physical activity (contributing approximately 200 kcal/day).

The ATP III report recommends that TLCs should be prescribed, with a vigorous emphasis on weight reduction and physical activity. Plasma LDL-C level should be lowered to ≤ 100 mg/dl. If TLC is not effective in 3–6 months, drug therapy is needed to lower LDL-C to the target of < 100 mg/dl. For high triglyceride levels (200–499 mg/dl) after these steps have been taken, non–HDL-C is recommended as a therapeutic target. The non–HDL-C goal is 30 mg/dl higher than the LDL-C goal. Non–HDL-C is obtained simply by subtracting the plasma level of HDL-C from the total cholesterol. Elevation > 130 mg/dl suggests elevation of LDL-C, and fibrate or nicotinic acid therapy is considered. In the case of an isolated low HDL-C levels in a diabetic, therapy with fibrates is recommended.

Key Points: Consensus for Intensive Management of Lipids and Lipoproteins in Type 2 Diabetes

- ∞ The ADA and the NCEP (ATP III) now agree in recommending intensive treatment for lipids/lipoproteins in type 2 diabetes.
- ∞ LDL-C is the primary target of therapy.
- ∞ Optimal levels of LDL-C are < 100 mg/dl.
- ∞ Triglycerides and HDL-C are secondary targets.
- ∞ Optimal triglyceride level is < 150 mg/dl.
- ∞ Optimal HDL-C levels are > 45 mg/dl for men and > 55 mg/dl for women.
- ∞ The first step is total lifestyle change (TLC).
- ∞ TLC includes a desirable body weight, exercise program, and meal plan with saturated fat < 7% of calories, cholesterol < 200 mg/day, and monounsaturated fat up to 20% of calories.
- ∞ TLC recommends 25–35% of calories as fat, 50–60% as carbohydrate, 15% as protein, and 20–30 gm of fiber daily.
- ∞ The non–HDL-C (cholesterol minus HDL-C) target is < 130 mg/dl. This goal should be used if high plasma triglyceride levels (200–499 mg/dl) are present after LDL-C is < 100 mg/dl.
- ∞ Fibrate or nicotinic acid therapy is recommended if the non–HDL-C level is > 130 mg/dl.

Evidence from Large-scale Randomized Trials for Intensive Management of Dyslipidemia in Type 2 Diabetes

LDL cholesterol

Lowering of LDL-C levels by statin therapy has been shown to lower the risk for major coronary events in primary and secondary prevention trials. Two primary prevention trials have been reported, primarily in nondiabetic subjects: the Air Force/Texas Coronary Atherosclerosis Prevention Study (AFCAPS/TEXCAPS)[53] and the West of Scotland Coronary Prevention Study (WOSCOPS).[184] The recently reported Heart Protection Study[22] is included in this group because about 46% of subjects at entry had no evidence of cardiovascular disease. Strictly speaking, however, it must be viewed as a mixed primary and secondary trial. Results of the three trials are summarized in Table 14.

It is apparent that statin therapy was associated with impressive cardiovascular risk reduction in these three trials. The results from the HPS are particularly impressive, since significant risk reductions were seen over the 5½ years of the study in a large subgroup of diabetics. A majority of this group (3982 = 67%) had no clinical evidence of prior coronary heart disease, and over 40% of the diabetic subjects had LDL-C levels < 115 mg/dl.[22] The 24% risk reduction was seen across all adult age groups in men and women with diabetes and at initial plasma cholesterol levels < 200 mg/dl and LDL-C concentrations < 120 mg/dl. This trial has provided the best evidence in support of a primary prevention strategy in type 2 diabetes and also provides strong support for an LDL-C goal of < 100 mg/dl or less.

There are two key secondary prevention trials of statin therapy in people with established coronary artery disease: the Cholesterol and Recurrent Events (CARE) Trial[38, 76] and the Scandinavian Simvastatin Survival Study (4S).[82, 83, 198] Both studies includes groups of diabetics large enough to provide subgroup analyses. Results from these trials are shown in Table 15.

The 4S population had higher LDL-C concentrations (187 mg/dl) than the CARE population (136 mg/dl). Mean LDL-C levels after statin therapy were 121 and 100 mg/dl, respectively. The CARE population did not have hypertriglyceridemia and were more likely to be revascular-

Table 14. Primary Prevention Trials of Statin Therapy					
Trial	No. Pts.	No. with Diabetes	Drug	↓ LDL-C	Results
AFCAPS-TEXCAPS	5068M 997F	155	Lovastatin	↓25%	37% reduction in risk for first coronary event, trend same in DM (NS)
WOSCOPS	6595M	76	Pravastatin	↓26%	31% reduction in risk for coronary event in DM (NS)
HPS	20,536	5963	Simvastatin	↓30%	≥ 24% reduction in risk for CV events in diabetic group (p < 0.001)

References for these trials are given in the text.

Table 15. Secondary Prevention Trials of Statin Therapy					
Trial	No. Pts.	No. with Diabetes	Drug	LDL-C	Results (DM)
CARE	3583 M 576 F	471 M 115 F	Pravastatin	↓27%	25% reduction in relative risk for major coronary events (p = 0.05)
4S	3617 M	483 M	Simvastatin	↓35%	42% reduction in risk for major coronary events (p = 0.001)

References for these trials are given in the text.

ized or treated with aspirin. These differences may explain the variations in magnitude of the cardiovascular risk reductions in the two trials.

From these five trials, it has been concluded that LDL-C–lowering with statin therapy is highly effective in diabetics and nondiabetics. Furthermore, in 4S a 38% reduction in the risk for major coronary events was seen in patients with impaired fasting glucose (110–125 mg/dl). At this stage, however, all of these results are from retrospective analyses of diabetic subgroups. They are subject, therefore, to potential bias and suffer from variable entry criteria and other clinical variables that may have altered results. For these reasons, primary and secondary prevention trials in predefined type 2 diabetic subjects, with major cardiovascular endpoints, are now under way. In the meantime, collective evidence supports a strategy of intensive LDL cholesterol-lowering in type 2 diabetes. Improved evidence-based definition of precise LDL-C targets are expected to emerge from these ongoing studies.

Triglycerides and HDL Cholesterol

There are three key prospective trials of fibrate therapy designed to lower plasma triglycerides and to raise HDL-C in nondiabetic and diabetic subjects: the Helsinki Heart Study,[116] the Veterans Affairs HDL Intervention Trial (VA-HIT),[171,179,180] and the Diabetes Atherosclerosis Intervention Study (DAIS).[190] Results are shown in Table 16.

These three trials of fibrate therapy show that it is effective in lowering elevated plasma triglyceride levels and in modestly raising HDL-C levels. Significant reduction in the rate of progression of angiographically proven CAD was shown in DAIS, and a significant reduction in coronary events occurred in VA-HIT, especially among patients with the metabolic syndrome. These significant results were supported by trends in the Helsinki Trial, in which the number of diabetic subjects was low. However, this trial included subjects with mixed dyslipidemia, many of whom presumably had the metabolic syndrome. Collectively, the three trials strongly support the recommendations for lifestyle and fibrate therapy as cardioprotective

	Table 16. Trials of Fibrate Therapy in Dyslipidemic Subjects						
Trial	Prevention	No. Pts.	No. with Diabetes	Drug	TG	LDL-C	Results
Helsinki	Primary (mixed dyslipidemia)	4081	135 M	Gemfibrozil	↓27%	↑5%	34% cor. events—total population. Trend for ↓ cor. events in DM (3.4%: gemfibrozil, 10.5%: placebo) NS
VA-HIT	Secondary	2531	627 M	Gemfibrozil	↓31%	↑6%	24% ↓ cor. events, stroke in DM (p = 0.05)
DAIS	Secondary	418	305 M 113 F	Fenofibrate	↓28%	↑6%	40% ↓ in rate of angiographic progression of CAD (p = 0.02)

References for these trials are given in the text.

strategies in people with metabolic syndrome and/or type 2 diabetes who have high plasma triglyceride and low HDL-C levels.

Intensive Management Strategies for Dyslipidemia

Effect of Glycemic Control on Lipoproteins

In type 2 diabetes, intensive glycemic control with nutrition therapy and an exercise program usually has a modest effect on plasma lipid and lipoprotein levels. A type 2 diabetic patient in poor metabolic control often does not meet therapeutic goals as far as lipoprotein metabolism is concerned, even after sulfonylurea therapy. In Table 17, the direction of the changes in lipids and lipoproteins in many people with type 2 diabetes is summarized after a period of poor vs. good control.[128]

Metformin and pioglitazone [100,128] may lower plasma triglyceride and raise HDL-C levels, but intensive therapeutic goals may not be reached,

Table 17. Effects of Glycemic Control on Lipids/Lipoproteins in Type 2 Diabetes		
Fasting Plasma Levels of Lipid/Lipoproteins	Poor Control	Good Control
Cholesterol	Increased	Normal or increased
Triglyceride	Markedly increased	Increased
VLDL	Markedly increased	Slightly increased
LDL-C	Increased	Normal
HDL-C	Markedly reduced	Reduced

even with combination therapy and good glycemic control. Drugs for lipid and lipoprotein regulation are often needed.

Drugs That Primarily Affect Lipoprotein Metabolism

Four main classes of drugs act primarily by affecting lipoprotein metabolism: HMGCoA reductase inhibitors (statins), bile acid sequestrants, nicotinic acid, and fibric acids (fibrates). Tables 18 and 19 summarize the range of therapeutic effects of these drugs on lipids and lipoproteins, their main side effects, contraindications to their use, and daily dosage.

Intensive Management Goals

LDL Cholesterol

Lowering of LDL-C is the primary goal, and levels are often above goal with intensive glucose control. The ADA has recommended stringent thresholds for the initiation of nutritional and pharmacologic therapy for LDL-C levels in patients with diabetes[12] (Table 20)

The NCEP(ATP III) guidelines are similar. In both cases, an LDL-C goal < 100 mg/dl is recommended. However, ATP III now considers a patient with type 2 diabetes as a CVD risk equivalent. With this designation, the distinction between diabetic patients with or without CHD, PVD, or CVD becomes irrelevant. Most type 2 diabetic patients with an LDL-C level above 100 mg/dl require statin therapy to achieve the goal

Table 18. Drugs That Affect Lipoprotein Metabolism			
Drug Class	**Effects on Lipid/Lipoproteins**	**Major Side Effects**	**Contraindications**
HMG CoA reductase inhibitors (statins)	LDL-C ↓ 18–55%	Myopathy, myalgia	Liver disease
	HDL-C ↑ 5–15%	Increased liver	Relative: concomitant
	TG ↓ 7–30%	Enzymes	use of certain drugs*
Bile acid sequestrants	LDL-C ↓ 15–30%	GI distress	TG > 400 mg/dl
	HDL-C ↑ 3–5%	Constipation	
	TG → or ↑	↓ Drug absorption	
Nicotinic acid	LDL-C ↓ 5–25%	Flushing	Liver disease
	HDL-C ↑ 15–35%	Hyperglycemia	Gout
	TG ↓ 20–50%	↑ uric acid	Relative: diabetes,
		Upper GI distress	hyperuricemia, peptic
		Hepatotoxicity	ulcer disease
Fibric acid (fibrates)	LDL-C ↓ 5–20%†	Dyspepsia	Severe renal disease
	HDL-C ↑ 10–20%	Myopathy	Liver disease
	TG ↓ 20–50%	Hepatotoxicity	

*Cyclosporine, macrolide antibiotics, antifungal agents, cytochrome P-450 inhibitors. Use fibrates and/or niacin with caution.
†LDL-C may rise in patients with high TG levels.

Table 19. Pharmacologic Agents Available in the U.S. for the Treatment of Lipids/Lipoproteins

Drug Class	Agent	Daily Dosage
HMG CoA reductase inhibitors (statins)	Atorvastatin	10–80 mg
	Fluvastatin	20–80 mg
	Lovastatin	10–40 mg
	Pravastatin	10–40 mg
	Simvastatin	10–80 mg
Bile acid sequestrants	Cholestyramine	4–16 gm
	Colestipol	5–20 gm
	Colesevelam	2.6–3.8 gm
Nicotinic acid	Niacin	1.5–3 gm
	Nicotinic acid (extended release)	1–2 gm
Fibric acid (fibrates)	Gemfibrozil	600 mg twice daily
	Fenofibrate	67–200 mg
	Clofibrate	1 gm twice daily

of < 100 mg/dl. Dose titration may be necessary, and the different preparations have dosage ranges that are usually effective in reaching the LDL-C goal. If the top dose of the chosen agent is ineffective, a shift to a more potent agent may be necessary. New statins with increasing effectiveness on lipids and lipoproteins are under study, and a wide range of choices is anticipated in future years.

Table 20. American Diabetes Association Thresholds for Initiation of Nutritional and Pharmacologic Therapy in Adults with Diabetes

Patient Characteristics	Medical Nutrition Therapy		Pharmacologic Therapy	
	Initiation Level	LDL-C Goal	Initiation Level	LDL-C Goal
With CHD, PVD, or CVD	> 100 mg/dl	≤ 100 mg/dl	> 100 mg/dL	≤ 100 mg/dl
Without CHD, PVD, or CVD	> 100 mg/dl	≤ 100 mg/dL	≥ 130 mg/dl	≤ 100 mg/dl

CHD = coronary heart disease, PVD = peripheral vascular disease, CVD = cardiovascular disease, LDL-C = low density lipoprotein cholesterol.
*For patients in borderline risk category (LDL-C between 100 and 129 mg/dl), strategies include more aggressive medical nutrition therapy and pharmacologic treatment with a statin.

Triglycerides and HDL-C

As noted in Table 18, the statins may also have favorable effects on plasma triglyceride and HDL-C levels. Because elevated triglycerides and low HDL-C levels are frequently present in the metabolic syndrome and type 2 diabetes, this effect is useful. Because the evidence is strong that elevated triglyceride levels and/or low plasma HDL-C concentrations are cardiovascular risk factors,[63] it is important to achieve designated therapeutic goals. Furthermore, as discussed previously, collaborative clinical trial evidence now supports the use of fibrates in lowering cardiovascular risk in type 2 diabetes with dyslipidemia. As is the case for LDL-C levels, there will be some improvement in altered triglyceride and/or HDL-C levels with intensive glycemic control (Table 17), but the goals of stringent management often are not met, even with intensive therapeutic lifestyle changes and multiple drug therapy for glycemia.

There is some disagreement between the ADA and the NCEP (ATP III) about goals for plasma triglyceride levels. The NCEP (ATIII) classification of triglyceride levels is as follows:

Normal	< 150 mg/dl
Borderline-high	150–199 mg/dl
High	200–499 mg/dl
Very high	≥ 500 mg/dl

The ADA agrees with the top two categories but classifies < 200 mg/dl as a desirable triglyceride level. The goal of therapy by ADA guidelines is to reduce fasting plasma triglyceride level to below 200 mg/dl. Prospective trial data (Table 16) indicate that a goal of < 150 mg/dl is preferable.

The NCEP (ATP III) points out that partially degraded VLDL (remnant lipoproteins) are atherogenic. In clinical practice, the VLDL cholesterol level is an estimate of these remnant lipoproteins. In persons with high plasma triglycerides (> 200 mg/dl), non–HDL-C is a secondary target for therapy. Non–HDL-C is calculated by subtracting HDL-C from total cholesterol. The non–HDL-C goal for people with type 2 diabetes is < 130 mg/dl.

An Approach to Intensive Lipid/Lipoprotein Management in Type 2 Diabetes

1. Draw blood after an overnight fast of at least 8 hours. Measure plasma levels of total cholesterol (TC), triglycerides (TG) and high-density lipoprotein cholesterol (HDL-C), and calculate low-density lipoprotein cholesterol (LDL-C).
2. Maximize glycemic control with medical nutrition therapy, weight loss, exercise, and drugs as required to achieve stable HbA1c values < 8%.
3. Monitor TC, TG, HDL-C, LDL-C quarterly if goals are not met; yearly if goals are met. The goals of therapy are as follows:
   - LDL-C < 100 mg/dl
   - TC < 200 mg/dl

- TG < 150 mg/dl
- HDL-C ≥ 45 mg/dl (men) ≥ 55 mg/dl (women)

4. If TC and LDL-C goals are not met, initiate statin therapy and raise the dosage quarterly until goals are achieved.
5. If TG goals are not met after LDL-C is < 100 mg/dl, add a fibrate. Monitor liver enzymes and creatine phosphokinase levels, and instruct patient about symptoms of myopathy.
6. This strategy often results in reaching TC, LDL-C, and TG goals without side effects. However, HDL-C levels often remain below normal. If non–HDL-C is < 130 mg/dl, no additional steps are needed.
7. Addition of niacin therapy to raise HDL-C and/or lower non–HDL-C is an option favored by some physicians. Evidence indicates that niacin-induced hyperglycemia can be managed.[56] If this option is chosen, careful monitoring for side effects of niacin, fibrates, and statins (Table 18) is clearly indicated.

Adherence to the Treatment Plan

The NCEP (ATP III) report gives useful guidelines (Table 21) to improve adherence to lipid/lipoprotein treatment plans. They are equally

---

Table 21. Interventions to Improve Adherence

1. Focus on the patient
   - Simplify medication regimens.
   - Provide explicit patient instruction and use good counseling techniques to teach the patient how to follow the prescribed treatment.
   - Encourage the use of prompts to help patients remember treatment regimens.
   - Use systems to reinforce adherence and maintain contact with the patient.
   - Reinforce and reward adherence.
   - Increase visits for patients unable to achieve treatment goal.
   - Increase the convenience and access to care.
   - Involve patients in their care through self-monitoring.
2. Focus on the physician and medical office
   - Teach physicians to implement lipid treatment guidelines.
   - Use reminders to prompt physicians to attend to lipid management.
   - Identify a patient advocate in the office to help deliver or prompt care.
   - Ask patients to promote preventive care.
   - Develop a standardized treatment plan to structure care.
   - Use feedback from past performance to foster change in future care.
   - Remind patients of appointments and follow-up missed appointments.
3. Focus on the health delivery system
   - Provide lipid management through a lipid clinic.
   - Utilize case management by nurses.
   - Deploy telemedicine.
   - Utilize the collaborative care of pharmacists.
   - Execute critical care pathways in hospitals.

applicable to intensive control of blood pressure or glycemic regulation in type 2 diabetes.

Key Points: Randomized Trial Evidence and Intensive Management of Dyslipidemia in Type 2 Diabetes

- ∞ Glycemic control improves the lipid profile in diabetic dyslipidemia but rarely returns plasma levels to normal.
- ∞ Three primary prevention trials have shown that a 25–30% reduction in LDL-C levels by statin therapy in type 2 diabetes leads to a 34–37% decrease in the risk for coronary events.
- ∞ Two secondary prevention trials have also shown impressive CV risk reduction by statin therapy in type 2 diabetics with CAD.
- ∞ Three prospective trials, primarily secondary prevention studies, have shown that lowering of TG by 27–31% and raising HDL-C by 5–6% with fibrate therapy decreases coronary events or angiographic progression of CAD in type 2 diabetes.
- ∞ The four classes of drugs available are the statins, bile acid sequestrants, nicotinic acid, and fibrates.
- ∞ An approach to intensive lipid/lipoprotein management in type 2 diabetes has been described (see pp 164–165).
- ∞ Interventions to improve adherence are of key importance for a successful program.

Procoagulant (Prothrombotic) State

Because vascular thrombosis is the major contributor to death in type 2 diabetes, there has been great interest in exploring the procoagulant (or prothrombotic) state in the disease.[45,46] Evidence supports the involvement of three systems in the procoagulant state:

- Intrinsic coagulation
- Fibrinolysis
- Platelets

Most studies have measured clotting factors, fibrinolytic components, and platelet function in a cross-section of typical type 2 diabetics. Good prospective trial evidence indicates antiplatelet agents are safe and effective in lowering the risk for cardiovascular events in people with type 2 diabetes. In regard to the other two systems, short-term studies indicate that favorable effects on a putative prothrombotic environment may be found with intensive glycemic treatment and therapy with certain drugs.[46]

Intrinsic Coagulation System

General activation of the intrinsic coagulation system has been described,[34] and Figure 4 indicates sites in the system that have been reported to be affected in type 2 diabetes. Activation of the system leads to the conversion of fibrinogen to the fibrin clot by the action of thrombin. Evidence indicates that factor VII and fibrinogen are cardiovascular risk factors in type 2 diabetes.

The plasma levels of some of these factors are affected by lowering of plasma glucose with insulin.[34,36] Generally, the changes are in the direction that would be expected to decrease the tendency for thrombosis. Thus, plasma fibrinogen levels correlate with the degree of blood glucose regulation and may fall with acutely administered insulin therapy in type 2 diabetes. HbA1c levels correlate with plasma levels of fibrinopeptide A and thrombin-antithrombin (TAT). Acute elevation of plasma glucose is accompanied by a rise in fibrinopeptide A and a fall in antithrombin III, and insulin infusion reverses these procoagulant changes.[34] Insulin administration lowers factor VII levels. Improved glycemic control has been

Figure 4. Pathways of blood coagulation. Circled are items that may be altered in diabetes. (−) = inhibitory effect; HMWK = high-molecular-weight kininogen; PF_3 = platelet factor 3; AT III = antithrombin III; HCIII = heparin cofactor III; α_2-MG, α_2-macroglobulin; FPA = fibrinopeptide A. (From Jokl R, Colwell JA: Clotting disorders in diabetes. In Alberti KGMM, Zimmet P, DeFronzo RA, et al (eds): International Textbook of Diabetes Mellitus, 2nd ed. Chichester, UK, John Wiley, 1997, pp 1543–1557; with permission.)

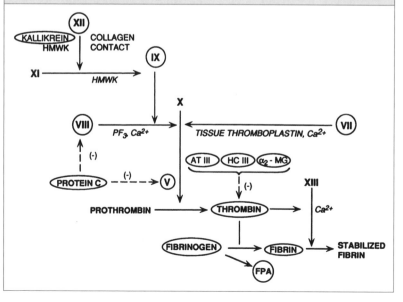

shown to reduce thrombus formation, as assessed in vitro using a perfusion chamber technique.[151]

There is little evidence from long-term prospective randomized trials in this area. The VA Cooperative Study in Type 2 Diabetes found a significant rise in mean plasma fibrinogen levels over baseline after 1 year in the group randomized to intensive insulin therapy.[57] Of interest, this short-term feasibility study also found a nonsignificant trend toward an increased incidence of cardiovascular events in the intensively treated group.[3] Intervention trials directed at plasma fibrinogen have been suggested.[35] Approaches to decrease plasma fibrinogen levels (and vascular risk) include cigarette smoking cessation, exercise programs, improved glycemic regulation, and use of drugs that decrease fibrinogen synthesis (e.g., ticlopidine, pentoxifylline, anabolic steroids, and fibrate drugs).

Fibrinolytic System

The fibrinolytic system maintains the patency of the vascular system. Plasmin is a proteolytic enzyme that acts to lyse fibrin deposits and thrombi. Plasminogen is a plasmin precursor that is converted to plasmin by the action of tissue plasminogen activator (tPA). Plasminogen activator inhibitor (PAI-1) is the major inhibitor of tPA. Thus, the balance between the activities of tPA and PAI-1 is critical in determining whether a fibrin clot is formed or whether it is lysed. It is hypothesized that elevated plasma levels of PAI-1 result in a prothrombotic state. The plasma PAI-1 level has been identified as a cardiovascular risk marker.[107]

Plasma PAI-1 levels are often elevated in type 2 diabetes and metabolic syndrome.[107,108] Levels correlate with plasma levels of triglycerides and insulin as well as with body mass index and centripetal obesity. Sources of plasma PAI-1 include visceral and subcutaneous adipose tissue,[7,59] vascular endothelium,[191] and the liver.[114] Of interest, approximately 90% of the total PAI-1 in humans is carried in the alpha granules of the blood platelets. Evidence indicates that PAI-1 is released by platelets after aggregation[105] and that it is physiologically active at the site of vascular injury to inhibit fibrinolysis and thereby promote thrombus formation.

Metabolic and hormonal control of PAI-1 synthesis and release has been described. High glucose concentrations increase transcription of the gene that codes for PAI-1 in human endothelial cell cultures. Synthesis of PAI-1 by cultured human hepatocytes is stimulated by insulin,[114] and proinsulin or insulin stimulates PAI-1 expression in bovine aortic endothelial cells. Endothelial release of PAI-1 is increased by oxidized or glycated low-density lipoproteins and very-low-density lipoproteins. Fig. 5 illustrates some of the postulated mechanisms for altered fibrinolytic activity in diabetes.

Acute exercise increases plasma fibrinolytic activity.[42,95] The effect in

Figure 5. Postulated mechanisms of altered fibrinolysis in diabetes. PAI-1 = plasminogen activator inhibitor-1; tPA = tissue plasminogen activator. (From Jokl R, Colwell JA: Clotting disorders in diabetes. In Alberti KGMM, Zimmet P, DeFronzo RA, et al (eds): International Textbook of Diabetes Mellitus, 2nd ed. Chichester, UK, John Wiley, 1997, pp 1543–1557; with permission.)

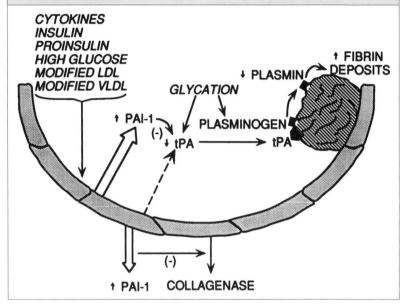

nondiabetics is seen immediately, and activity is correlated with the intensity and duration of the exercise. This increase in fibrinolysis correlates with a fall of PAI-1 levels. However, effects of exercise on fibrinolysis are absent or less robust in people with type 2 diabetes compared with nondiabetic subjects. Plasma PAI-1 levels decrease with acute and chronic weight loss in obese people.[37,137] People with the highest plasma PAI-1 and triglyceride levels are the most responsive. A provocative study of type 2 diabetics found that a low glycemic index diet was associated with a 54% fall in plasma PAI-1 levels to normal.[103] This effect was not seen in the group given a high glycemic index diet and was not explained by a difference in weight reduction in the two groups. Thus, it appears that exercise conditioning, weight loss, and a diet low in glycemic index decrease plasma PAI-1 levels in type 2 diabetes.

Oral antidiabetic agents also have been shown to affect this system. Metformin has been shown to increase fibrinolytic activity in people with coronary artery disease[17,18] and lowers plasma PAI-1 levels in type 2 diabetics.[145] This effect is maintained for at least 36 months and is seen at doses as low as 1500 mg/day.[77] Troglitazone therapy is associated with a fall in PAI-1 levels in women with polycystic ovary syndrome[55] and in type 2 diabetes.[62,117] Similar results have been reported with the newer thiazolidinediones, pioglitazone and rosiglitazone.[67] An elevated plasma PAI-1 level is now considered by many to be a component of metabolic syndrome. It is postulated that insulin sensitizers reduce PAI-1 levels by lowering insulin resistance, decreasing plasma triglyceride and/or free fatty acid levels, and lowering plasma levels of insulin and/or proinsulin In contrast to metformin and the thiazolidinediones, sulfonylureas have no effect on plasma PAI-1 levels in type 2 diabetes, and insulin administration has no consistent effect.

Other agents may decrease elevated plasma PAI-1 levels. Lowering of elevated plasma triglyceride levels by gemfibrozil has been associated with a fall in plasma PAI-1 levels. It has been recently recognized that the renin-angiotensin system is involved in regulating fibrinolytic balance.[210] Angiotensin II increases PAI-1 production, and ACE inhibition lowers plasma PAI-1 levels after myocardial infarction. ACE inhibitor therapy with fosinopril lowers plasma PAI-1 levels in type 2 diabetes compared with the calcium channel blocker amlodipine.[152] Finally, in postmenopausal women, conjugated estrogens alone or in combination with progestational agents reduce plasma PAI-1 antigen levels by 50%.[113]

There are a number of promising leads for therapy directed at altered fibrinolysis in type 2 diabetes. Monitoring of plasma PAI-1 is now under way in a number of prospective randomized trials in type 2 diabetes, and correlation with cardiovascular events is a major goal. Table 22 summarizes the effects of nutrition therapy, exercise, and drugs on plasma PAI-1 levels.

Table 22. Effect of Nutrition Therapy, Exercise and Drugs on Plasma PAI-1 Levels in Type 2 Diabetes	
Therapy	**Effect on Plasma PAI-1 Level**
Weight reduction	Decrease
Low glycemic index diet	Decrease
Physical training	Decrease
Metformin	Decrease
Thiazolidinediones	Decrease
Gemfibrozil	Decrease*
ACE inhibitors	Decrease
Estrogens/progestins	Decrease†
Sulfonylureas	No effect
Insulin	No effect

*If triglyceride level is increased.
†In post menopausal women.

Platelets

The many alterations of platelet function reported in type 2 diabetes are summarized in Table 23. The increased activity of the thromboxane production system has been the major target for chronic therapy because of the sensitivity of the platelet cyclooxygenase enzyme to inhibition by low doses of aspirin. Increased platelet thromboxane release has been described in type 1[85] and type 2[49] diabetes. Cyclooxygenase catalyzes the conversion of arachidonic acid to prostaglandins G2 and H2, precursors to thromboxane. This arachidonic acid metabolite is a potent vasoconstrictor and a platelet proaggregant. The inhibition of thromboxane production is immediate and lasts throughout the lifespan of the platelets (about 10 days). Each day new platelets enter the bloodstream at a rate of about 10%/day, and repeated daily doses of as little as 40 mg of aspirin irreversibly inhibit the cyclooxygenase of new platelets. Clinically, aspirin is prescribed in doses of 81–325 mg/day for inhibition of thromboxane synthesis. Ibuprofen (400 mg) blocks this effect of aspirin when given directly before aspirin ingestion or even if it is prescribed three times daily on a regular basis. Acetaminophen and diclofenac do not have this effect.[32] Cycolooxygenase-2 inhibitors do not affect aspirin's action and can be used if clinically indicated (e.g., for arthritis). Larger doses of aspirin are effective but carry increased risk of gastrointestinal or central nervous system bleeding. Enteric coating is believed to decrease gastrointestinal irritation and does not inhibit efficacy. Prospective trials have shown that aspirin therapy does not carry an increased risk of retinal, vitreous, or central nervous system bleeding when hypertension is controlled. An increase in the risk for minor gastrointestinal bleeding is the main side effect of chronic aspirin therapy.

Primary, mixed primary, and secondary prevention trials that have supported the use of aspirin in people with type 2 diabetes are summarized in Table 24. Primarily as a result of these studies, the ADA has recommended

Table 23. Alterations of Platelet Function in Diabetes	
Increased	**Decreased**
Platelet aggregability	Nitric oxide production
Arachidonic acid metabolism	Antioxidant levels
Thromboxane synthesis	Membrane fluidity
Platelet—plasma interactions (immune complexes, glycated LDL)	Intracellular magnesium-to-calcium ratio
Adhesion molecule expression (glycoprotein IIb/IIIa, P-selectin)	
Platelet adhesiveness	
Storage and release of PAI-1	

Table 24. Use of Aspirin in Diabetes						
Study	Primary or Secondary Prevention	Endpoints	% of Patients with Event		Relative Risk	p
			Aspirin	Placebo		
Physicians' Health Study[189]	Primary	Total myocardial infarction	4.0	10.1	0.39	‡
Early Treatment Diabetic Retinopathy Study[194]	Mixed	Myocardial infarction	9.1	12.3	0.83	0.03
Hypertension Optimal Treatment[87]	Mixed†	Major cardiovascular events	8.9*	10.5*	0.85	0.03
		Myocardial infarction	2.3*	3.6*	0.64	0.002
Antiplatelet Trialists' Collaboration[15]	Secondary	Vascular events	18.5	22.3	0.75	0.002

*Events/1000 patient-years.
†All: diastolic blood pressure 100–115 mmHg
‡Not reported.

that enteric coated aspirin, 81–325 mg/day, should be used as preventive therapy in diabetic men and women over age 30 who are at high risk for a cardiovascular event.[8,40] Recommendations are given in Table 25.

In a study of type 2 diabetics in the Third National Health and Nutrition Examination Survey (NHANES III), 27% were eligible for aspirin therapy as secondary prevention and an additional 71% had one or more predictors of cardiovascular events.[172] Thus, virtually every type 2 diabetic in the U.S. is eligible for aspirin therapy under ADA guidelines. However, only 13% of those with one or more risk factors received this simple, safe, inexpensive form of therapy at the time of the NHANES III study.

Alternatives to aspirin are also effective. Clopidogrel and ticlopidine inhibit platelet function by pathways district from the arachidonic acid to thromboxane route. These compounds inhibit adenosine diphosphate binding to its platelet receptor and thereby prevent activation of the glycoprotein IIb/IIIa receptor. This, in turn, inhibits fibrinogen binding, and platelet adhesiveness is diminished. In one large study of nondiabetics and diabetics (Clopidogrel vs. aspirin in Patients at Risk of Ischemic Events [CAPRIE]),[31] clopidogrel (75 mg/day) was slightly superior to aspirin (325 mg/day) in preventing ischemic stroke, myocardial infarction, or vascular death (5.32% vs 5.83%, $p < 0.032$). Ticlopidine has been shown to decrease the rate of microaneurysm progression in type 1 and type 2 diabetics with nonproliferative diabetic retinopathy.[199] The side effect of severe neutropenia in 2–4% of patients limits the use of ticlopidine. Clopidogrel does not have this side effect and is recommended as an alternative to aspirin in patients who cannot take aspirin.

Table 25. Recommendations for Aspirin Therapy in People with Diabetes

1. Use aspirin therapy as a secondary prevention strategy in diabetic men and women who have evidence of large vessel disease. This includes diabetic men and women with a history of myocardial infarction, vascular bypass procedure, stroke or transient ischemic attack, peripheral vascular disease, claudication, and/or angina.
2. In addition to treating the primary cardiovascular risk factor(s) identified, consider aspirin therapy as a primary prevention strategy in high-risk men and women with type 1 or type 2 diabetes. This includes diabetics with the following risk factors.
   - A family history of coronary heart disease
   - Cigarette smoking
   - Hypertension
   - Overweight/obesity ($>$ 120% desirable weight): BMI $>$ 27.3 in women or $>$ 27.8 in men
   - Albuminuria (micro or macro)
   - Lipids
     Cholesterol $>$ 200 mg/dl
     LDL cholesterol $>$ 100 mg/dl
     HDL cholesterol $<$ 45 mg/dl in men and $<$ 55 mg/dl in women
     Triglycerides $>$ 200 mg/dl
   - Age $>$ 30 years
3. Use enteric-coated aspirin in doses of 81–325 mg/day.
4. People with aspirin allergy, bleeding tendency, anticoagulant therapy, recent gastrointestinal bleeding, and clinically active hepatic disease are not candidates for aspirin therapy.
5. Use of aspirin has not been studied in diabetics under the age of 30 years. Aspirin therapy should not be recommended for patients under the age of 21 years because of the increased risk of Reye's syndrome associated with aspirin use in this population.

Limited studies of the effects of oral antidiabetic agents or insulin on platelet function indicate that these agents may decrease platelet aggregation and/or thromboxane release, probably as a result of greatly improved glycemic control.[45,122]

Key Points: Procoagulant (Prothrombotic) State

- A prothrombotic state is often present in type 2 diabetes.
- Three systems are affected in type 2 diabetes: intrinsic coagulation, fibrinolysis, and platelets.
- Type 2 diabetes is associated with general activation of the intrinsic coagulation system.
- Two components of this system, factor VII and fibrinogen, have been found to be cardiovascular risk factors.
- In general, improved glycemic regulation with insulin changes intrinsic coagulation factors in a direction that would decrease the tendency for thrombosis.
- An inhibitor of clot lysis, PAI-1, is present in excess in many people with metabolic syndrome, type 2 diabetes, and/or obesity.

Key Points (*Continued*)

- Ninety percent of the PAI-1 in the body is carried in blood platelets.
- Elevated plasma PAI-1 levels are lowered by weight reduction, physical training, low glycemic index diets, and various drugs, including metformin, thiazolidinediones, gemfibrozil (if triglyceride levels are high), ACE inhibitors, and estrogens/progestins in menopausal women.
- There are many alterations of platelet function in diabetes, including increased adhesiveness, aggregability, and thromboxane synthesis.
- Four trials (primary and secondary) have shown that aspirin decreases cardiovascular events (primarily myocardial infarction) in type 2 diabetes.
- No increased risk of retinal, vitreous, or central nervous system bleeding was seen in these controlled trials.
- From 81 to 325 mg of enteric-coated aspirin should be given to all type 2 diabetics who are at high risk for cardiovascular disease. Studies indicate that this constitutes 98% of the U.S. population with type 2 diabetes.

Congestive Heart Failure

Epidemiologic Data

The Framingham Study first showed over 20 years ago an increased risk of congestive heart failure (CHF) in patients with diabetes.[109] Recent advances in the medical and surgical management of coronary heart disease have increased survival rates. Coronary heart disease has now replaced hypertension and valvular heart disease as the primary cause of CHF.[50] The incidence of CHF after a myocardial infarction is doubled in people with type 2 diabetes and is a major contributor to increased mortality and morbidity.

A recent longitudinal study in 9591 people with type 2 diabetes compared prevalence and incidence rates of CHF to an age- and sex-matched control group without diabetes.[147] CHF was found in 11.8% of diabetic subjects and 4.5% of control subjects at baseline. Over 30 months, the incidence of CHF in subjects who did not have CHF at baseline was 7.7% in type 2 diabetics and 3.4% in controls. Thus, close to 20% of people with type 2 diabetes in this large prospective study had CHF. Independent risk factors for CHF in diabetes included age, diabetes duration, insulin use, ischemic heart disease, and elevated serum creatinine. The slopes of increasing prevalence and incidence of CHF across age groups were similar in those with or without diabetes. Better glycemic control at baseline and improved glycemic and blood pressure control at follow-up predicted the development of CHF. Insulin use was associated with CHF after adjustment for other variables. No data about thiazolidinediones were available. Because of possible fluid retention, these agents should not be used in patients with NYHA class III or IV CHF.

This study dramatically illustrates the problem of CHF in type 2 diabetes. An interesting finding was the association with insulin use and improved glycemic control. Similar CHF trends were seen in the VA Feasibility Study.[3] The findings emphasize the need for further study of the effects of intensive glycemic management with insulin and insulin sensitizers on CHF. These studies are presently under way in the VA- and NIH-sponsored randomized trials of intensive vs. standard glycemic management in type 2 diabetes.

Management of CHF in type 2 diabetes is clearly an important issue. In addition to the usual approaches with sodium restriction and loop diuretics, evidence indicates that ACE inhibitor therapy and beta receptor blockade are effective.

ACE Inhibitors

A number of collaborative trials support the use of ACE inhibitor therapy in CHF. In meta-analysis of 34 completed trials, patients with CHF (ejection fractions of 45% or less), Garg et al. concluded that total mortality and hospitalization for CHF were significantly reduced by ACE inhibitor therapy.[70] There was a statistically significant reduction in total mortality, with an odds ratio of 0.65 (p < 0.001). Effects were most prominent in the first 5 months of therapy, and patients with the lowest ejection fraction had the greatest benefit. Results were applicable to a wide range of patients. Full ACE inhibitor doses were usually needed. Angiotensin receptor blockers were less effective and were used as second-line therapy in 20% of patients (e.g., those who developed ACE inhibitor cough).

Beta Receptor Blockade

An overview of randomized controlled clinical trials of second- and third-generation beta blockers in patients with NYHA class II–IV heart failure has been reported.[64] In more than 10,000 patients, it was found that beta blockers reduced mortality and morbidity. Reduction in mortality risk ranged from 35–65% in four trials with significant findings. Meta-analyses have concluded that the use of beta blockers is associated with a consistent 30% reduction in mortality and a 40% reduction in hospitalizations in patients with heart failure.[64] Guidelines for patient selection and procedures for using beta blockers in heart failure have been developed.[61]

Results appear to apply to diabetic and nondiabetic patients. One study with an analysis of results in diabetic patients is the Metoprolol CR/XL Randomized Intervention Trial in Congestive Heart Failure (MERITCHF).[92] This trial showed that beta blockade with metroprolol CR/XL (titrated upward to the full dosage of 200 mg/day) improved survival, reduced hospitalizations for CHF, and improved NYHA functional class. The study includes 3991 patients with chronic CHF, NYHA functional class II–IV, and ejection fraction of 40% or less. There was a 31% risk reduction in total mortality or hospitalizations due to worsening CHF. A subgroup of 977 people with diabetes had a similar risk reduction in total mortality or hospitalization for CHF when metroprolol CR/XL was compared with placebo.

As a result of these and other trials, ACE inhibitor therapy now has multiple indications in people with type 2 diabetes, and beta blocker therapy, which was previously discouraged in diabetics, is now indicated in the presence of CHF and after an acute myocardial infarction. The benefits clearly outweigh the minimal risks of changes in plasma lipids or loss of recognition of symptoms of hypoglycemia. Furosemide is used in addition to ACE inhibitor and beta blocker therapy. In the event that left ventricular function, as estimated by ejection fraction, returns to 60% or more, the consensus is to decrease the furosemide dosage slowly and to continue ACE inhibitor and beta blocker therapy indefinitely. Finally, a walking program has been shown to increase exercise capacity and quality of life for people with CHF.

Multiple Risk Factors

The Metabolic Syndrome

In 1988, in his Banting Lecture before the ADA, Reaven described syndrome X as a condition characterized by (1) resistance to insulin-stimulated glucose uptake, (2) glucose intolerance, (3) hyperinsulinemia, (4) increased very-low-density lipoprotein triglyceride, (5) decreased high-density lipoprotein cholesterol, and (6) hypertension.[163] He suggested that this cluster of abnormalities contributed to the 2- to 4-fold increased risk in people with diabetes for atherothrombotic vascular disease. Subsequently, the syndrome has been called the insulin resistance syndrome and, most recently, metabolic syndrome. A recent focused definition from the National Cholesterol Education Program (Adult Treatment Panel III) is given in Table 26.[60] The World Health Organization includes microalbuminuria in the definition, and many observers add a prothrombotic state since increased plasma levels of PAI-1, fibrinogen, and/or factor VII may be present.

Meigs et al. used factor analysis to determine whether insulin resistance is a single process that underlies the clustering of the classic risk factors of the syndrome.[138] They concluded that three independent processes were involved: (1) a central metabolic syndrome of hyperin-

Table 26. Characteristics of the Insulin Resistance Syndrome (Metabolic Syndrome)[60]		
Abdominal obesity		
Waist circumference	> 40 inches (males)	
	> 35 inches (females)	
Fasting plasma triglycerides ≥ 150 mg/dl		
Fasting plasma HDL cholesterol		
	< 40 mg/dl (males)	
	< 50 mg/dl (females)	
Blood pressure ≥ 130/85 mmHg		
Fasting plasma glucose ≥ 110 mg/dl		
(3 or more of these must be present for the diagnosis of metabolic syndrome)		

sulinemia, dyslipidemia, and obesity; (2) glucose intolerance; and (3) hypertension. Glucose intolerance and hypertension are linked to the central syndrome by hyperinsulinemia and obesity. Similarly, it has been impossible to separate the individual contributions of insulin resistance, hyperglycemia, dyslipidemia, and the procoagulant state to the accelerated atherosclerosis and thrombosis of diabetes (Fig. 6)

The metabolic syndrome, as defined in the NCEP (ATP III) report, was

Figure 6. One interpretation of insulin resistance syndrome. Three distinct physiologic domains combine to form the insulin resistance syndrome: central metabolic syndrome (high correlation of encircled risk variables with factor 1), impaired glucose tolerance (factor 2), and hypertension (factor 3). The domains are linked by neutral associations with hyperinsulinemia (reflecting insulin resistance) and obesity. (From Meigs JB et al. Diabetes 46:1594–1600, 1997, with permission.)

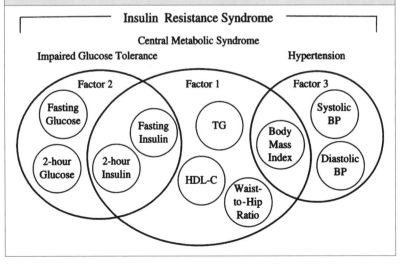

frequently found among adults in the U.S. who were enrolled in 1988–1994 in the NHANES III Study.[66] The age-adjusted prevalence was 23.7% among 8814 men and women aged 20 years or older. Prevalence increased from 6.7% (ages 20–29) to 43.5% (ages 60–69). The syndrome was more prevalent in African American and Mexican American women than in men. Using the 2000 census data, about 47 million U.S. residents are estimated to have the metabolic syndrome.

Metabolic syndrome has a high prevalence in multiple large population studies around the world.[25,132,181] Of interest, a recent large study in Finland and Sweden found that 10–15% of males and females with normal glucose tolerance, 42–64% with impaired fasting glucose or impaired glucose tolerance, and 74–84% with type 2 diabetes had two or more components of this syndrome.[102] Cardiovascular mortality in patients with metabolic syndrome was 12.0% vs 2.2% in controls (p < 0.0001) over a median follow-up time of 6.9 years. Thus, metabolic syndrome is quite common in type 2 diabetes in many populations and is often present in people with impaired fasting glucose or impaired glucose tolerance. Aggressive risk factor reduction strategies are indicated for this large cohort of people at extremely high risk for cardiovascular events.

Key Points: Metabolic Syndrome

- ᴄ⨀ Other names are syndrome X and the insulin resistance syndrome.
- ᴄ⨀ It is estimated that 47 million people in the U.S. have metabolic syndrome.
- ᴄ⨀ Approximately 10–15% of people with normal glucose tolerance, 42–64% of those with IGT, and 74–84% with type 2 diabetes have two or more components of metabolic syndrome.
- ᴄ⨀ Cardiovascular mortality is increased 5-fold in people with metabolic syndrome.
- ᴄ⨀ Components of the metabolic syndrome include:
  1. Abdominal obesity
  2. Fasting plasma values (mg/dl): TG ≥ 150; HDL-C < 40 (men) or < 50 (women); glucose ≥ 110; increased levels of small dense LDL-C
  3. Microalbuminuria: > 30 mg albumin/24-hr urine
  4. Hypertension: BP ≥ 130/85 mm Hg
  5. Prothrombotic state: increased levels of PAI-1, factor VII, fibrinogen
- ᴄ⨀ Early identification of people with metabolic syndrome and intensive risk factor therapeutic strategies are critical issues for health professionals to implement.

ACE Inhibitor Therapy in Type 2 Diabetes

Heart Outcomes Prevention Evaluation (HOPE) Trial

The HOPE Trial enrolled 9297 people with a history of coronary or peripheral vascular disease or diabetes.[90,196,197] Of these 3577 diabetics were defined as high risk by virtue of a previous cardiovascular event, hypertension (BP of 160/90 mmHg or treatment), albuminuria (> 30 mg urinary albumin/24 hr), cholesterol > 200 mg/dl, HDL cholesterol <40 mg/dl, or cigarette smoking.[90] Subjects were randomized to receive an ACE inhibitor (ramipril 10 mg) or placebo. They were followed for 4.5 years. In this worldwide study, 50% of patients were from Canada and only 10% from the U.S. The mean age was 66 ± 7 years, and 73% of patients were men.

A 24% reduction in the risk for the combined endpoint of myocardial infarction, stroke, or cardiovascular disease-related death was seen in the diabetic group (p < 0.001). Analyses of the effect of ACE inhibitor therapy on individual cardiovascular endpoints also showed a significant risk reduction (Table 27). All of these risk reductions were significant at the level of p < 0.01. In the diabetic subgroup, ramipril reduced the risk of a combined microvascular outcome of overt nephropathy, dialysis, or laser therapy by 16% (p = 0.036). Fewer subjects on ramipril therapy (102) developed a new diagnosis of diabetes compared with placebo (155); the relative risk was 0.66 (p < 0.001).

Should we generalize from this study and recommend that virtually all patients with type 2 diabetes be placed on ACE inhibitor therapy? Epidemiologic analyses of the NHANES III type 2 diabetic cohort showed that 98% had at least one other cardiovascular risk factor. Thus, in the United States, virtually all type 2 diabetics may have been candidates for this trial. However, 90% of the HOPE study participants were from outside the U.S., and no ethnic breakdown was given in the report. The ethnic mix in the U.S. includes substantial numbers of African Americans, Hispanics, and Asians. About two-thirds of the HOPE study diabetic population had

Table 27. Cardiovascular Risk Reductions in the HOPE Study and in the Diabetic Group[90,196,197]		
	Total Study (n = 9297)	Diabetes (n = 3578)
Primary endpoint*	21%	24%
Myocardial Infarct	20%	22%
Stroke	31%	33%
Cardiovascular death	25%	37%
Total mortality	16%	24%
*Myocardial infarction, stroke, or cardiovascular death.		

evidence of preexisting cardiovascular disease—a very high ratio. One can conclude, however, that elderly Caucasian type 2 diabetic patients with previous cardiovascular disease, hypertension, microalbuminuria, elevated cholesterol level, or low HDL cholesterol level should be considered for ACE inhibitor therapy. This conclusion substantially expands older criteria for ACE inhibitor therapy in diabetes. Other studies support this view in diabetic subjects with the complications of albuminuria, hypertension, heart failure, or recent myocardial infarction.

What are the mechanisms for the protective effects leading to a decreased progression of retinopathy or nephropathy? Exploration of mechanisms was not a primary goal of the HOPE trial, but one can speculate, based on previous studies of the actions of ACE inhibitors. Was protection in the ramipril group due to the small but measurable reduction in blood pressure (3.3/1.9 mmHg), which exceeded that seen with placebo? Intuitively, this effect seems unlikely to account for all of the vascular protection. However, the recently reported Hypertension Outcomes Trial[87,88] showed that minimal differences in degree of reduction of diastolic blood pressure by antihypertensive agents had a significant cardiovascular risk reduction in diabetics with hypertension.

Other mechanisms are also likely. Angiotensin II (AII) has many vascular actions, including vasoconstriction, promotion of vascular smooth muscle cell proliferation, decreased endothelial function, and decreased fibrinolytic activity. Evidence indicates an increased local activation of the renin angiotensin system within the blood vessels in the diabetic state. AII may potentiate the action of the sympathetic nervous system and activate free radical formation in vascular walls. Thus, one can theorize a number of actions of AII that were presumably blocked by ACE inhibitor therapy to contribute to the significant decrease in cardiovascular events.

What about the effects on the microcirculation of the retina or kidney? Studies of a renoprotective action of ACE inhibitor therapy in type 1 and type 2 diabetes are described in other sections. Thus, several studies have shown that ACE inhibitor therapy decreases albumin excretion rate and progression of renal insufficiency in people with diabetes and albuminuria. Biopsy evidence suggests a decrease in glomular damage after ACE inhibitor therapy vs. placebo in type 1 diabetes. It is likely that the reduction of the rate of progression of diabetic retinopathy by ACE inhibitor therapy was due to inhibition of the action of AII to stimulate the expression of vascular endothelial growth factor (VEGF) in vascular smooth muscle. VEGF may stimulate cytokines that lead to angiogenesis and increased vascular permeability of retinal microvessels. The blood pressure decline of approximately 3/2 mmHg may have played a role. The findings that ACE inhibitor therapy resulted in a decrease in progression of retinopathy are in agreement with the EURODIAB Controlled Trial of Lisinopril in Insulin-dependent Diabetes (EUCLID), in which lisinopril was associated with a decrease in progression of retinopathy (vs. placebo) in normotensive type 1 diabetic subjects.[195]

Could the results be explained by an improvement in glycemic regulation during the study? The UKPDS showed a significant risk reduction in progression of diabetic retinopathy and nephropathy in the group of people with type 2 diabetes randomized to an intensive management strategy, with mean HbA1c 0.9% below that of the control group (7.0 vs 7.9%). Improved glycemic regulation was not seen in the HOPE trial, for the ramipril group had a calculated baseline HbA1c of 7.4%, which rose to 9.6% by the end of the study. Of great interest, cardioprotective and microcirculatory protective results were seen with HbA1c levels well in excess of current ADA guidelines at the conclusion of the study.

Why should ACE inhibitor therapy delay progression from the nondiabetic to the diabetic state? This intriguing finding may be related to the vasoconstrictive action of AII. Studies clearly show that ACE inhibitor therapy leads to a decrease in insulin resistance as well as an increase in pancreatic insulin secretion. Either or both of these effects may be mediated by an increased microcirculatory flow in muscle and/or pancreatic islets. The latter effect has clearly been shown in elegant in vivo studies in a rat model, and increased insulin sensitivity with ACE inhibitor has been demonstrated by in vivo glucose-insulin clamp studies in humans.

Finally, in this cost-conscious climate it is refreshing to note evidence from other studies that treatment of people with diabetes over the age of 50 with ACE inhibitor drugs is less expensive than screening first for gross proteinuria and compares favorably with the costs of screening first for microalbuminuria before initiating therapy.[75]

As a result of this accumulating body of evidence, we may see much wider use of ACE inhibitor therapy in people with diabetes who are at high cardiovascular risk and in nondiabetics who have had a previous cardiovascular event.

Homocysteine

For many years it has been recognized that people who inherit a genetic deficiency in the metabolism of homocysteine, an amino acid derived from the metabolism of methionine, have markedly accelerated cardiovascular disease. Acquired hyperhomocysteinemia may occur in the presence of deficiencies of folate, pyridoxine (B_6), and vitamin B_{12}. It has been reported that people with type 1 diabetes, particularly those with albuminuria and/or renal failure, may have elevated plasma homocysteine levels.[41,93] Epidemiologic information indicates that the relative risk for cardiovascular disease is more than doubled among people with plasma homocysteine levels in the top 20% of the population.[212] These levels are usually greater than 13 μmol/L. Risk increases progressively along the spectrum of homocysteine levels, and homocysteine remains a significant risk factor when blood pressure and apolipoprotein B levels are taken into account.

Studies in a group of patients with type 1 diabetes of at least 10 years' duration have shown that 35% had elevated plasma homocysteine levels.[41] In the majority, this elevation was seen in the fasting state. Vascular complications were more frequent in this group, suggesting that homocysteine may have contributed to accelerated vascular disease. High levels were particularly common in the presence of microalbuminuria (30–300 mg albumin excretion/24 hours), clinical albuminuria (> 300 mg albumin excretion/24 hours), and renal failure.

Studies are limited in patients with type 2 diabetes, but two studies have shown a correlation of plasma homocysteine levels and cardiovascular disease in a type 2 population.[94,144] Many studies have shown elevated plasma homocysteine levels in the presence of renal insufficiency of any cause.[214] Some evidence suggests that plasma homocysteine levels, microalbuminuria, and hyperinsulinemia occur in metabolic syndrome. Elevated plasma homocysteine levels have been reported in poorly controlled type 2 diabetic patients, but not in adolescents with type 1 diabetes.[157]

Short-term studies have shown that an increase in folic acid intake can decrease elevated plasma homocysteine levels. Although results from randomized collaborative trials are pending about the impact of this therapy on cardiovascular disease, it has been estimated that fortification of food with folic acid could prevent 13,500–50,000 deaths due to coronary artery disease in the U.S. each year. Vitamin B_6 (pyridoxine) should be added to normalize abnormal methionine metabolism from homocysteine. Vitamin B_{12} is also recommended to avoid the issue of B_{12} neuropathy in folic acid-treated patients. For these reasons, some physicians treat patients with elevated fasting plasma homocysteine levels with these three vitamins. Usual doses are between 1.0 and 5.0 mg of folic acid, 10–50 mg of vitamin B_6, and up to 1 mg/day of vitamin B_{12}.

It therefore appears reasonable to add homocysteine to the list of vascular risk factors in people with diabetes and to consider vitamin supplementation in high-risk patients with high homocysteine levels. Often these patients have a decrease in glomerular filtration rate due to diabetic nephropathy.

C-Reactive Protein

Highly sensitive assays have established that the plasma level of C-reactive protein (CRP) is a marker of atherosclerosis.[89,118,139,168,169] Studies by Ross have postulated that atherosclerosis is as an inflammatory disease.[176] Inflammatory macrophages, T lymphocytes, cytokines, and adhesion molecules appear to interact with endothelium and smooth muscle cells in the pathogenesis of early atherosclerotic lesions. Lipid-laden macrophages form fatty streaks, and a fibrous cap forms over proliferated smooth muscle, mitogens, inflammatory cells, and intra- and extracellular lipids. Plaques may become vulnerable to rupture, and inflammatory cells predominate at sites of rupture. Vascular thrombosis may then occur.

CRP is an acute-phase reactant produced by the liver in response to inflammatory stimuli.[158] An elevated plasma CRP level is a marker of inflammation. In view of the inflammation theory of pathogenesis of atherosclerosis, many studies have focused on the role of CRP in vascular disease. Population studies have shown an association of plasma CRP levels and coronary artery disease (CAD).

Prospective studies have indicated that the CRP level is a predictor of cardiovascular mortality and morbidity. Thus, in the CARE Trial, baseline elevation of CRP was predictive of higher risk for recurrent cardiovascular events.[170] In the Multiple Risk Factor Intervention Trial (MRFIT), the baseline CRP level had a correlation with CAD mortality among smokers. In the Physicians Health Study (PHS), participants with higher CRP levels at baseline had significantly higher risk for cardiovascular events than those with normal CRP levels.[168] Similar findings emerged from the Women's Health Study.[159,169] In most studies, the predictive value of CRP persisted after controlling for possible confounders (e.g., smoking, lipids, diabetes).

Recent work has indicated that plasma CRP levels are elevated in people with centripetal obesity, insulin resistance, and type 2 diabetes.[68] Plasma levels of CRP rise as a function of BMI. In one study, 26–51% of people with BMI > 30 kg/m^2 had elevated plasma CRP levels.[43,65] Levels are higher in people with impaired fasting glucose or diabetes than in nondiabetic matched subjects. In this study, 34–39% of patients with diabetes had elevated plasma CRP levels. As yet, there are no longitudinal studies in people with metabolic syndrome or diabetes to give insight into the possible sequence of events. It may be postulated that insulin resistance is the common denominator in people with excess body weight or type 2 diabetes. Studies have shown that tumor necrosis factor alpha (TNFα) and interleukin-6 (IL-6) levels are elevated in both insulin-resistant states.[159,221] TNFα and IL-6 may stimulate the expression of adhesion molecules in the vasculature, and this response may be followed by smooth muscle cell proliferation and endothelial permeability. Both are early signs of arterial damage. In diabetes, advanced glycation products may stimulate macrophages and lymphocytes to secrete cytokines. Abdominal adipose tissue is a source of IL-6, and the cytokines IL-1 and IL-6 act on the liver to increase production of acute-phase reactants, including CRP. The end result may be an increase in blood viscosity, activation of the intrinsic coagulation system, increased platelet adherence and/or aggregability, and/or inhibition of lysis of the fibrin clot. There is even evidence in animals that the acute-phase response is associated with increase in plasma VLDL and a decrease in HDL cholesterol. Thus, one can correlate many aspects of atherosclerosis and thrombosis with the increased acute-phase reaction in obesity, type 2 diabetes, and metabolic syndrome.

The good news is that CRP has clinical utility, because preventive interventional approaches appear to be successful. However, newly developed, highly sensitive assays are needed rather than the older CRP assay traditionally used in clinical laboratories. Low-dose aspirin therapy (325 mg every other day) led to a 44% risk reduction for the first myocardial infarction in the PHS,[168] and efficacy improved in patients with diabetes and in people with elevated levels of CRP. In the CARE Trial, pravastatin therapy resulted in a greater risk reduction (54%) in patients with elevated CRP than in those without elevation (25%).[170]

Thus plasma CRP levels may be elevated, using the highly sensitive assay, in people with metabolic syndrome and/or type 2 diabetes. If these findings reflect atherosclerosis of an inflammatory nature, additional studies of prevention of cardiovascular events by agents such as aspirin and statins in these syndromes would be of interest. Furthermore, the statins have multiple antiatherothrombotic properties.[174] The effectiveness of aspirin therapy in preventing cardiovascular events has been demonstrated in studies such as the Hypertension Optimal Treatment (HOT) Trial[87] and the Early Treatment of Diabetic Retinopathy Study (ETDRS).[194] Measurement of plasma CRP by the highly sensitive CRP assay in type 2 diabetes may identify a group of patients who are candidates for aspirin or statin therapy; however, additional long-term primary prevention trials in diabetic subjects and those at risk for developing diabetes are needed to explore this postulate.

Key Points: Congestive Heart Failure and Multiple Risk Factors in Type 2 Diabetes

- CHF is more prevalent in type 2 diabetes than in age and gender matched controls.
- In one study, about 20% of type 2 patients had CHF vs. 8% of control subjects.
- Good evidence indicates that CHF in diabetes should be treated with ACE inhibitors and cardiospecific beta receptor blockade in addition to diuretic therapy.

Key Points (*Continued*)

∞ The HOPE Trial has shown that type 2 diabetics with high cardiovascular risk have a 22–37% reduction in risk with ACE inhibitor therapy.

∞ ACE inhibitor therapy may delay progression from the nondiabetic to the diabetic state in people who have high cardiovascular risk.

∞ Plasma homocysteine level is a cardiovascular risk factor.

∞ About 35% of people with diabetes of ≥ 10 years' duration have elevated plasma homocysteine levels.

∞ Levels are usually elevated in patients with renal insufficiency.

∞ Folic acid, pyridoxine, and vitamin B_{12} therapy lower elevated plasma homocysteine levels, but prospective trials are needed to determine whether this treatment reduces cardiovascular events.

∞ Plasma CRP levels determined by a new, highly sensitive assay may be elevated in obesity and type 2 diabetes.

∞ CRP is a marker of inflammation and atherosclerosis. When the sensitive assay is used, plasma CRP level is a predictor of cardiovascular mortality and morbidity.

∞ Collaborative trial evidence indicates that aspirin and statins lower CRP levels and cardiovascular events.

References

1. A Joint Editorial Statement by the American Diabetes Association; the National Heart, Lung and Blood Institute; the Juvenile Diabetes Foundation International: the National Institute of Diabetes and Digestive and Kidney Diseases; and the American Heart Association: Diabetes mellitus: A major risk factor for cardiovascular disease. Circulation 100:1132–1133, 1999.

2. A study of the effects of hypoglycemic agents on vascular complications in patients with adult-onset diabetes: 11. Mortality results, University Group Diabetes Program. Diabetes 19(Suppl. 2):789–830, 1970.

3. Abraira C, Colwell J, Nuttall F, et al: Cardiovascular events and correlates in the Veterans Affairs Diabetes Feasibility Trial. Veterans Affairs Cooperative Study on Glycemic Control and Complications in Type 2 Diabetes. Arch Intern Med 157:181–188, 1997.

4. Abraira C, Colwell JA, Nuttall FQ, et al: Veterans Affairs Cooperative Study on Glycemic Control and Complications in Type II Diabetes (VA CSDM): Diabetes Care 18:1113–1123, 1995.

5. Abraira C, Henderson WG, Colwell JA, et al: Response to intensive therapy steps and to glipizide dose in combination with insulin in type 2 diabetes. VA feasibility study on glycemic control and complications (VA CSDM). Diabetes Care 21:574–579, 1998.

6. Ajani UA, Gaziano M, Lotufo PA, et al: Alcohol consumption and risk of coronary heart disease by diabetes status. Circulation 102:500–505, 2000.

7. Alessi MC, Peiretti F, Morange P, et al: Production of plasminogen activator inhibitor 1 by human adipose tissue: Possible link between visceral fat accumulation and vascular disease. Diabetes 46:860–867, 1997.

8. American Diabetes Association: Aspirin therapy in diabetes. Diabetes Care 25:S78–S79, 2002.

9. American Diabetes Association: Diabetes mellitus and exercise. Diabetes Care 25:S64–S68, 2002.

10. American Diabetes Association: Diabetic nephropathy. Diabetes Care 25:S85–S89, 2002.

11. American Diabetes Association: Evidence-based nutrition principles and recommendations for the treatment and prevention of diabetes and related complications. Diabetes Care 25:S50–S60, 2002.

12. American Diabetes Association: Management of dyslipidemia in adults with diabetes. Diabetes Care 25:S74–S77, 2002.

13. American Diabetes Association: Standards of medical care for patients with diabetes mellitus. Diabetes Care 25:S33–S49, 2002.

14. American Diabetes Association: Treatment of hypertension in adults with diabetes. Diabetes Care 25:S71–S73, 2002.

15. Antiplatelet Trialists' Collaboration: Collaborative overview of randomised trials of antiplatelet therapy, I: Prevention of death, myocardial infarction, and stroke by prolonged antiplatelet therapy in various categories of patients. BMJ 308:81–106, 1994.

16. Aviles-Santa L, Sinding J, Raskin P: Effects of metformin in patients with poorly controlled, insulin-treated type 2 diabetes mellitus: A randomized, double-blind, placebo-controlled trial. Ann Intern Med 131:182–188, 1999.

17. Bailey CJ: Biguanides and NIDDM. Diabetes Care 15:755–772, 1992.

18. Bailey CJ, Turner, RC: Drug therapy: Metformin. N Engl J Med 334:574–579, 1996.

19. Bakau B, Shipley M, Jarrett RJ, et al: High blood glucose concentration is a risk factor for mortality in middle-aged nondiabetic men. 20-year follow-up in the Whitehall Study the Paris Prospective Study, and the Helsinki Policemen Study. Diabetes Care 21:360–367, 1998.

20. Bakris G, Weston WM, Rappaport EB, et al: Rosiglitazone produces long-term reductions in urinary albumin excretion in type 2 diabetes. Diabetologia 42(Suppl 1):230A, 1999.

21. Bakris GL, Williams M, Dworkin L, et al: Special Report: Preserving renal function in adults with hypertension and diabetes: A consensus approach. Am J Kidney Dis 36:646–661, 2000.

22. Collins R, Armitage J, Parish S, et al: MRC/BHF heart protection study of cholesterol lowering with simvastatin in 20,536 high-risk individuals: A randomized placebo-controlled trial. Lancet 360:7–22, 2002.

23. Bastyr EJ III, Stuart CA, Brodows RG, et al, for the IOEZ Study Group: Therapy focused on lowering postprandial glucose, not fasting glucose, may be superior for lowering HbA1c. Diabetes Care 23:1236–1241, 2000.

24. Beks PHJ, Mackaay AJC, de Vries H, et al: Carotid artery stenosis is related to blood glucose level in an elderly Caucasian population: The Hoorn Study. Diabetologia 40:290–298, 1997.

25. Bonora E, Kiechl S, Willeit J, et al. Prevalence of insulin resistance in metabolic disorders: the Bruneck Study. Diabetes 47:1643–1649, 1998.

26. Boucher JL, Shafer KJ, Chaffin, JA: Weight loss, diets, and supplements: Does anything work? Diabetes Spectr 14:169–175, 2001.

27. Boulé NG, Haddad E, Kenny GP, et al: Effects of exercise on glycemic control and body mass in type 2 diabetes mellitus. A meta-analysis of controlled clinical trials. JAMA 286:1218–1227, 2001.

28. Brenner BM: Hemodynamically mediated glomerular injury and the progressive nature of kidney disease. Kidney Int 23:647–655, 1983.

29. Brenner BM, Cooper ME, De Zeeuw D, et al: Effects of losartan on renal and car-

diovascular outcomes in patients with type 2 diabetes and nephropathy. N Engl J Med 345:861–869, 2001.

30. Campbell IW, Howlett HCS: Worldwide experience of metformin as an effective glucose-lowering agent: A meta-analysis. Diabetes Metab Rev 11:S57–S62, 1995.

31. CAPRIE Steering Committee: A randomised, blinded, trial of clopidogrel versus aspirin in patients at risk of ischaemic events (CAPRIE). Lancet 348:1329–1339, 1996.

32. Catella-Lawson F, Reilly MP, Kapoor SC, et al: Cyclooxygenase inhibitors and the antiplatelet effects of aspirin. N Engl J Med 345:1809–1817, 2001.

33. Cefalu WT, Skyler JS, Kourides IA, et al. Inhaled human insulin treatment in patients with type II diabetes mellitus. Ann Intern Med 134:203–207, 2001.

34. Ceriello A: Coagulation activation in diabetes mellitus: The role of hyperglycaemia and therapeutic prospects. Diabetologia 36:1119–1125, 1993.

35. Ceriello A: Fibrinogen and diabetes mellitus: Is it time for intervention trial? Diabetologia 40:731–734, 1997.

36. Ceriello A, Giugliano D, Quatraro A, et al: Evidence for a hyperglycaemia-dependent decrease of antithrombin III-thrombin complex formation in humans. Diabetologia 33:163–167, 1990.

37. Charles MA, Morange P, Eschwege E, et al: Effect of weight change and metformin on fibrinolysis and the von Willebrand factor in obese nondiabetic subjects: The BIGPRO1 Study. Biguanides and the Prevention of the Risk of Obesity. Diabetes Care 21:1967–1972, 1998.

38. Cholesterol and Recurrent Events (CARE) Trial Investigators: The effect of pravastatin on coronary events after myocardial infarction in patients with average cholesterol levels. N Engl J Med 335:1001–1009, 1996.

39. Collins AR, Meehan WP, Kintscher U, et al: Troglitazone inhibits formation of early atherosclerotic lesions in diabetic and nondiabetic low density lipoprotein receptor-deficient mice. Arterioscler Thromb Vasc Biol 21:365–371, 2001.

40. Colwell JA: Aspirin Therapy in Diabetes (Position Statement). Diabetes Care 20:1772–1773, 1997.

41. Colwell JA: Elevated plasma homocysteine and diabetic vascular disease [editorial]. Diabetes Care 20:1805–1806, 1997.

42. Colwell JA: Effects of exercise on platelet function, coagulation, and fibrinolysis. Diabetes Metab Rev 1:501–512, 1986.

43. Colwell JA: Inflammation and diabetic vascular complications [editorial]. Diabetes Care 22:1927–1928, 1999.

44. Colwell JA: Is it time to introduce metformin in the U.S.? Diabetes Care 16:653–655, 1993.

45. Colwell JA: Treatment for the procoagulant state in type 2 diabetes. Endocrinol Metab Clin North Am 30:1011–1030, 2001.

46. Colwell JA, Jokl: Vascular thrombosis in diabetes. In: Porte D, Sherwin R, Rifkin H, eds. Diabetes Mellitus: Theory and Practice, 5th ed. Norwalk, CT, Appleton & Lange 1996, pp 207–216.

47. Coutinho M, Gerstein HC, Wang YM et al: The relationship between glucose and incident cardiovascular events: a metaregression analysis of published date from 20 studies of 95,783 individuals followed for12.4 years. Diabetes Care 22:233–240, 1999.

48. Curb JD, Pressel SL, Cutler JA, et al: Effect of diuretic-based antihypertensive treatment on cardiovascular disease risk in older diabetic patients with isolated systolic hypertension. JAMA 276:1886–1892, 1996.

49. Davi G, Belvedere M, Vigneri S, et al: Influence of metabolic control on thromboxane biosynthesis and plasma plasminogen activator inhibitor type 1 in non-insulin-dependent diabetes mellitus. Thromb Haemost 76:34–37, 1996.

50. Davis RC, Hobbs FDR, Lip GYH: ABC of heart failure: history and epidemiology. BMJ 320:39–42, 2000.

51. DeFronzo RA, Goodman AM: Efficacy of metformin in patients with non-insulin-dependent diabetes mellitus. N Engl J Med 333:541–549, 1995.

52. Diabetes Prevention Program Research Group: Reduction in the incidence of Type 2 diabetes with lifestyle intervention or metformin. N Engl J Med 346:393–403, 2002.

53. Downs JR, Clearfield M, Weiss S, et al, for the AFCAPS/TexCAPS Research Group: Primary prevention of acute coronary events with lovastatin in men and women with average cholesterol levels: results of AFCAPS/TexCAPS. JAMA 279:1615–1622, 1998.

54. Edelman D, Edwards LJ, Olsen MK, et al. Screening for diabetes in an outpatient clinic population. J Gen Intern Med 17:23–28, 2002.

55. Ehrmann DA, Schneider DJ, Sobel BE, et al: Troglitazone improves defects in insulin action, insulin secretion, ovarian steroidogenesis, and fibrinolysis in women with polycystic ovary syndrome. J Clin Endocrinol Metab 82:2108–2116, 1997.

56. Elam MB, Hunninghake DB, Davis KB, et al: Effect of niacin on lipid and lipoprotein levels and glycemic control in patients with diabetes and peripheral arterial disease. The ADMIT Study: A randomized trial. JAMA 284, 1263–1270, 2000.

57. Emanuele N, Azad N, Abraira C, et al: Effect of intensive glycemic control on fibrinogen, lipids, and lipoproteins. Arch Intern Med 158:2485–2490, 1998.

58. Epstein M, Sowers JR: Diabetes mellitus and hypertension. Hypertension 19:403–418, 1992.

59. Eriksson P, Reynisdottir S, Lonnqvist F, et al: Adipose tissue secretion of plasminogen activator inhibitor-1 in non-obese and obese individuals. Diabetologia 41:65–71, 1998.

60. Executive Summary of the Third Report of the National Cholesterol Education Program (NCEP) Expert Panel on Detection, Evaluation, and Treatment of High Blood Cholesterol in Adults (Adult Treatment Panel III). JAMA 285:2486–2497, 2001.

61. Farrell MH, Foody JM, Krumholz HG: β-blockers in heart failure. Clinical applications. JAMA 287:890–897, 2002.

62. Fonseca VA, Reynolds T, Hemphill D, et al: Effect of troglitazone on fibrinolysis and activated coagulation in patients with non-insulin-dependent diabetes mellitus. J Diabetes Compl 12:181–186, 1998.

63. Fontbonne A, Eschwege E, Cambien F: Hypertriglyceridemia as a risk factor of coronary heart disease mortality in subjects with impaired glucose tolerance or diabetes: results from the 11-year follow-up of the Paris Prospective Study. Diabetologia 32:300–304, 1989.

64. Foody JM, Farrell MH, Krumholz HM: β-blocker therapy in heart failure. Scientific review. JAMA 287:883–889, 2002.

65. Ford ES: Body mass index, diabetes, and C-reactive protein among U.S. adults. Diabetes Care 22:1971–1977, 1999.

66. Ford ES, Giles WH, Dietz WH, et al: Prevalence of the metabolic syndrome among US adults. Findings from the third national health and nutrition examination survey. JAMA 287:356–359, 2002.

67. Freed M, Fuell D, Menci L, et al: Effect of combination therapy with rosiglitazone and glibenclamide on PAI-1 antigen, PAI-1 antigen, PAI-1 activity, and tPA in patients with type 2 diabetes [abstract]. Diabetologia 32:1024, 2000.

68. Frohlich M, Imhof A, Berg G, et al. Association between C-reactive protein and features of the metabolic syndrome: a population-based study. Diabetes Care 23:1835–1839, 2000.

69. Gaede P, Vedel P, Parving HH, et al: Intensified multifactorial intervention in patients with type 2 diabetes mellitus and microalbuminuria: the Steno type 2 randomised study. Lancet 353:617–622, 1999.

70. Garg R, Yusuf S, for the Collaborative Group on ACE Inhibitor Trials: Overview of randomized trials of angiotensin-converting enzyme inhibitors on mortality and morbidity in patients with heart failure. JAMA 273:1450–1456, 1995.

71. Geiss LS, Rolka DB, Engelgau MM: Elevated blood pressure among U.S. adults with diabetes, 1988–1994. Am J Prev Med 22:42–48, 2002.

72. Gillow JT, Gibson JM, Dodson PM: Hypertension and diabetic retinopathy—what's the story: Br J Ophthalmol 83:1083–1087, 1999.

73. Giugliano D, Quatraro A, Consoli G, et al: Metformin for obese, insulin-treated diabetic patients: Improvement in glycaemic control and reduction of metabolic risk factors. Eur J Clin Pharmacol 50:107–112, 1993.

74. Glass CK: Anti-atherogenic effects of thiazolidinediones: Arterioscler Thromb Vasc Biol 21:295–296, 2001.

75. Golan L, Birkmeyer JD, Welch HG: The cost-effectiveness of treating all patients with type 2 diabetes with angiotensin-converting enzyme inhibitors. Ann Intern Med 131:660–667, 1999.

76. Goldberg RB, Mellies MJ, Sacks FM: Cardiovascular events and their reduction with pravastatin in diabetic and glucose-intolerant myocardial infarction survivors with average cholesterol levels. Subgroup analyses in the cholesterol and recurrent events (CARE) Trial. Circulation 98:2513–2519, 1998.

77. Grant PJ: The effects of high- and medium-dose metformin therapy on cardiovascular risk factors in patients with type 2 diabetes. Diabetes Care 19:64–66, 1996.

78. Groeneveld Y, Patri H, Hermans J, et al. Relationship between blood glucose level and mortality in type 2 diabetes mellitus: a systematic review. Diabetes Med 116:2–13, 1999.

79. Gu K, Cowie CC, Harris MI: Diabetes and decline in heart disease mortality in US adults. JAMA 281:1291–1297, 1999.

80. Gu K, Cowie CC, Harris MI: Mortality in adults with and without diabetes in a national cohort of the U.S. population, 1971–1993. Diabetes Care 21:1138–1145, 1998.

81. Guay DRP: Repaglinide, a novel, short-acting hypoglycemic agent for type 2 diabetes mellitus. Pharmacotherapy 18:1195–1204, 1998.

82. Haffner SM: The scandinavian simvastatin survival study (4S) subgroup analysis of diabetic subjects: Implications for the prevention of coronary heart disease. Diabetes Care 20:469–471, 1997.

83. Haffner SM, Alexander CM, Cook TJ, et al: Reduced coronary events in simvastatin-treated patients with coronary heart disease and diabetes or impaired fasting glucose levels. Arch Intern Med 159:2661–2667, 1999.

84. Haffner SM, Lehto S, Ronnemaa T, et al: Mortality from coronary heart disease in subjects with type 2 diabetes and in nondiabetic subjects with and without prior myocardial infarction. N Engl J Med 339:229–234, 1998.

85. Halushka PV, Rogers RC, Loadholt CB, et al: Increased platelet thromboxane synthesis in diabetes mellitus. J Lab Clin Med 97:87–96, 1981.

86. Hanefeld M, Dickinson S, Bouter KP, et al: Rapid and short-acting mealtime insulin secretion with nateglinide controls both prandial and mean glycemia. Diabetes Care 23:202–207, 2000.

87. Hansson L, Zanchetti A, Carruthers SG, et al: Effects of intensive blood-pressure lowering and low-dose aspirin in patients with hypertension: principal results of the Hypertension Optimal Treatment (HOT) randomised trial. Lancet 351:1755–1762, 1998.

88. Hansson L, Zanchetti A for the HOT Study Group: The Hypertension Optimal Treatment (HOT) Study-Patient characteristics: randomization , risk profiles, and early blood pressure results Blood Press 3:322–327, 1994.

89. Haverkate F, Thompson SG, Pyke SD, et al: Production of C-reactive protein and risk

of coronary events in stable and unstable angina: European Concerted Action on Thrombosis and Disabilities Angina Pectoris Study Group. Lancet 349:462–466, 1997.

90. Heart Outcomes Prevention Evaluation (HOPE) Study Investigators: Effects of ramipril on cardiovascular and microvascular outcomes in people with diabetes mellitus: Results of the HOPE study and MICRO-HOPE substudy. Lancet 355:253–259, 2000.

91. Henry RR, Gumbiner B. Ditzler T, et al: Intensive conventional insulin therapy for type 2 diabetes.: Metabolic effects during a 6 month outpatient trial. Diabetes Care 16:21–27, 1993.

92. Hjalmarson A, Goldstein S, Fagerberg B, et al: Effects of controlled-release metoprolol on total mortality, hospitalizations, and well-being in patients with heart failure. The metoprolol CR/XL randomized intervention trial in congestive heart failure (MERIT-CHF). JAMA 283:1295–1302, 2000.

93. Hofmann MA, Kohl B, Zumbach MS, et al: Hyperhomocyste(e)inemia and endothelial dysfunction in IDDM. Diabetes Care 20:1880–1886, 1997.

94. Hoogeveen EK, Kostense PJ, Beks PJ, et al: Hyperhomocysteinemia is associated with an increased risk of cardiovascular disease, especially in non-insulin-dependent diabetes mellitus: a population-based study. Arterioscler Thromb Vasc Biol 18:133–138, 1998.

95. Hornsby WG, Boggess KA, Lyons TJ, et al: Hemostatic alterations with exercise conditioning in NIDDM. Diabetes Care 13:87–92, 1990.

96. Hostetter TH: Prevention of end-stage renal disease due to type 2 diabetes. [Editorial] N Engl J Med 345:910–911, 2001.

97. Hu S, Wang S, Dunning BE: Tissue selectivity of antidiabetic agent nateglinide: Study on cardiovascular and beta-cell KATP channels. J Pharmacol Exp Ther 291:1372–1379, 1999.

98. Hu S, Wang S, Fanelli B, et al: Pancreatic β-cell KATP channel activity and membrane-binding studies with nateglinide: A comparison with sulfonylureas and repaglinide. J Pharmacol Exp Ther 293:444–452, 2000.

99. Imano E, Kanda T, Nakatani Y, et al: Effect of troglitazone on microalbuminuria in patients with incipient diabetic nephropathy. Diabetes Care 21:2135–2139, 1998.

100. Inzucchi SE: Oral antihyperglycemic therapy for type 2 diabetes. JAMA 287:360–372, 2002.

101. Inzucchi SE, Maggs DG, Spollett GR, et al: Efficacy and metabolic effects of metformin and troglitazone in type 2 diabetes mellitus. N Engl J Med 338:867–872, 1998.

102. Isomaa B, Almbfen P, Tuomi T, et al: Cardiovascular morbidity and mortality associated with the metabolic syndrome. Diabetes Care 24:683–689, 2001.

103. Jarvi AE, Karlstrom BE, Granfeldt YE, et al: Improved glycemic control and lipid profile and normalized fibrinolytic activity on a low-glycemic index diet in type 2 diabetic patients. Diabetes Care 22:10–18, 1999.

104. Johnson JL, Wolf SL, Kabadi UM: Efficacy of insulin and sulfonylurea combination therapy in type II diabetes. Arch Intern Med 156:259–264, 1996.

105. Jokl R, Klein RL, Lopes-Virella MF, et al: Release of platelet plasminogen activator inhibitor 1 in whole blood is increased in patients with type 2 diabetes. Diabetes Care 18:1150–1155, 1995.

106. Jovanovic L, Dailey G III, Huang W-C, et al: Repaglinide in type 2 diabetes: A 24-week fixed-dose efficacy and safety study. J Clin Pharmacol 40:49–57, 2000.

107. Juhan-Vague I, Alessi MC, Vague P: Increased plasma plasminogen activator inhibitor-1 levels: A possible link between insulin resistance and atherothrombosis. Diabetologia 34:457–462, 1991.

108. Juhan-Vague I, Roul C, Alessi MC, et al: Increased plasminogen activator inhibitor activity in non-insulin dependent diabetic patients—relationship with plasma insulin. Thromb Haemost 3:370–373, 1989.

109. Kannel WB, McGee DL: Diabetes and cardiovascular disease: the Framingham study. JAMA 241:2035–2038, 1979.

110. Keilson L, Mather S, Walter YH, et al: Synergistic effects of nateglinide and meal administration on insulin secretion in patients with type 2 diabetes mellitus. J Clin Endocrinol Metab 85:1081–1086, 2000.

111. Khaw KT, Wareham N, Luben R, et al: Glycated haemoglobin, diabetes, and mortality in men in Norfolk cohort of European Prospective Investigation of Cancer and Nutrition (EPIC-Norfolk). BMJ 322:15–18, 2001.

112. Klein R: Hyperglycemia and microvascular and macrovascular disease in diabetes. Diabetes Care 18:258–268, 1995.

113. Koh KK, Mincemoyer R, Bui MN, et al: Effects of hormone-replacement therapy on fibrinolysis in postmenopausal women. N Engl J Med 336:683–690, 1997.

114. Kooistra T, Boma PJ, Tons HA, et al: Plasminogen activator inhibitor 1: Biosynthesis and mRNA level are increased by insulin in cultured human hepatocytes. Thromb Haemost 62:723–728, 1989.

115. Koshiyama H, Shimono D, Kuwamura N, et al. Inhibitory effect of pioglitazone on carotid arterial wall thickness in type 2 diabetes. J Clin Endocrinol Metab 86:3452–3456, 2001.

116. Koskinen P, Manttari M, Manninen V, et al: Coronary heart disease incidence in NIDDM patients in the Helsinki study. Diabetes Care 15:820–825, 1992.

117. Kruszynska YT, Yu JG, Olefsky JM, et al: Effects of troglitazone on blood concentrations of plasminogen activator inhibitor 1 in patients with type 2 diabetes and in lean and obese normal subjects. Diabetes 49:633–639, 2000.

118. Kuller LH, Tracy RP, Shaten J, et al: Relation of c-reactive protein and coronary heart disease in the MRFIT nested case-control study. Am J Epidemiol 144:537–547, 1996.

119. Kuusisto J, Mykkanen L, Pyorala K, et al: NIDDM and its metabolic control predict coronary heart disease in elderly subjects. Diabetes 43:960–967, 1994.

120. Laakso M: Perspective in Diabetes. Hyperglycemia and cardiovascular disease in Type 2 diabetes. Diabetes 48:937–942, 1999.

121. Laakso M, Rannemaa T, Pyorala K, et al: Atherosclerotic vascular disease and its risk factors in non-insulin-dependent and non-diabetic subjects in Finland. Diabetes Care 11:449–463, 1988.

122. Larkins RG, Jerums G, Taft JL, et al: Lack of effect of gliclazide on platelet aggregation in insulin-treated and non-insulin-treated diabetes: A two-year controlled study. Diabetes Res Clin Pract 4:81–87, 1988.

123. Lauer MS, Fontanarosa PB: Updated guidelines for cholesterol management. JAMA 285:2508–2509, 2001.

124. Law RE, Meehan WP, Zi XP, et al: Troglitazone inhibits vascular smooth muscle cell growth and intimal hyperplasia. J Clin Invest 98:1897–1905, 1996.

125. Lebovitz HE: Alpha-glucosidase inhibitors as agents in the treatment of diabetes. Diabetes Rev 6:132–145, 1998.

126. Lebovitz HE, Banerji MA: Insulin resistance and its treatment by thiazolidinediones. Recent Prog Horm Res 56:265–294, 2001.

127. Lebovitz HE: Insulin secretogogues: Old and new. Diabetes Rev 7:139–153, 1999.

128. Lebovitz HE: Oral therapies for diabetic hyperglycemia. Endocrinol Metab Clin North Am 30:909–933, 2001.

129. Lepore M, Pampanelli S, Fanelli C, et al: Pharmacokinetics and pharmacodynamics of subcutaneous injection of long-acting human insulin analog glargine, NPH insulin, and ultralente human insulin and continuous subcutaneous infusion of insulin lispro. Diabetes 49:2142–2148, 2000.

130. Lewis EJ, Hunsicker LG, Clarke WR, et al: Renoprotective effect of the angiotensin-receptor antagonist irbesartan in patients with nephropathy due to type 2 diabetes. N Engl J Med 345:851–860, 2001.

131. Lewis E, Hunsicker L, Bain R, et al: The effect of angiotensin-converting-enzyme inhibition on diabetic nephropathy. N Engl J Med 329:1456–1462, 1993.

132. Liese AD, Mayer-Davis EJ, Tyroler HA, et al: Development of the multiple metabolic syndrome in the ARIC cohort: joint contribution of insulin, BMI, and WHR. Ann Epidemiol 7:407–416, 1997.

133. Lopes-Virella MF, Stone PG, Colwell JA. Serum high density lipoprotein in diabetic patients. Diabetologia 13:285–291, 1977.

134. Maggio CA, Pi-Sunyer FX: The prevention and treatment of obesity. Application to type 2 diabetes. Diabetes Care 20:1744–1766, 1997.

135. Malmberg K, Rydén L, Efendic S, et al: Randomized trial of insulin-glucose infusion followed by subcutaneous insulin treatment in diabetic patients with acute myocardial infarction (DIGAMI Study): Effects on mortality at 1 year. J Am Coll Cardiol 26:57–65, 1995.

136. Malmberg K for the DIGAMI (Diabetes Mellitus, Insulin Glucose Infusion in Acute Myocardial Infarction) Study Group. Prospective randomised study of intensive insulin treatment on long term survival after acute myocardial infarction in patients with diabetes mellitus. BMJ 314:1512–1515, 1997.

137. Mehrabjian M, Peter JB, Barnard RJ, et al: Dietary regulation of fibrinolytic factors. Atherosclerosis 84:25–32, 1990.

138. Meigs JB, D'Agostino RB Sr, Wilson PW et al: Risk variable clustering in the insulin resistance syndrome: The Framingham Offspring Study. Diabetes 46:1594–1600, 1997.

139. Mendall MA, Patel P, Ballam L, et al: C-reactive protein and its relation to cardiovascular risk factors: a population based cross sectional study. BMJ 312:1061–1065, 1996.

140. Minamikawa J, Tanaka S, Yamauchi M, et al: Potent inhibitory effect of troglitazone on carotid arterial wall thickness in type 2 diabetes. J Clin Endocrinol Metab 83:1818–1820, 1998.

141. Mogensen CE, Neldam S, Tikkanen I, et al: Combination therapy with candesartan and lisinopril was more effective than monotherapy in type 2 diabetes and hypertension. BMJ 321:1440–1444, 2000.

142. Mudaliar S, Edelman SV: Insulin therapy in Type 2 diabetes. Endocrinol Metab Clin North Am 30:935–979, 2001.

143. Mudaliar S, Henry RR: New oral therapies for type 2 diabetes mellitus: The glitazones or insulin sensitizers. Annu Rev Med 52:239–257, 2001.

144. Munshi MN, Stone A, Fink L, Fonseca V: Hyperhomocysteinemia following a methionine load in patients with non-insulin-dependent diabetes mellitus and macrovascular disease. Metabolism 45:133–135, 1996.

145. Nagi DK, Yudkin JS: Effects of metformin on insulin resistance, risk factors for cardiovascular disease, and plasminogen activator inhibitor in NIDDM subjects: A study of two ethnic groups. Diabetes Care 16:621–629, 1993.

146. Nathan D, et al: Inhaled insulin for type 2 diabetes: Solution or Distraction? [editorial]. Ann Intern Med 134:242–244, 2001.

147. Nichols GA, Hillier TA, Erbey JR, et al: Congestive heart failure in type 2 diabetes. Prevalence, incidence, and risk factors. Diabetes Care 24:1614–1619, 2001.

148. Nielsen FS, Rossing P, Gall MA, et al: Long-term effect of lisinopril and atenolol on kidney function in hypertensive NIDDM subjects with diabetic nephropathy. Diabetes 46:1182–1188, 1997.

149. Ohkubo Y, Kishikawa H, Araki E, et al: Intensive insulin therapy prevents the progression of diabetic microvascular complications in Japanese patients with non-insulin-dependent diabetes mellitus: a randomized prospective 6-year study. Diabetes Res Clin Pract 28:103–117, 1995.

150. Orloff DG, Blazine MA, O'Connor CM: Atherosclerotic disease in non-insulin-dependent diabetes mellitus: Role of abnormal lipids and the place for lipid-altering therapies. Am Heart J 138:S406–S412, 1999.

151. Ounde JI, Badimon JJ, Fuster V, et al: Blood thrombogenicity in type 2 diabetes patients is associated with glycemic control. J Am Coll Cardiol 38:1307–1312, 2001.

152. Pahor M, Franse LV, Deitcher SR, et al: The fosinopril versus amlodipine comparative treatments study (FACTS), a randomized trial to assess drug effects on PAI-1. Circulation 102:417–418, 2000.

153. Parker B, Noakes M, Luscombe N, Clifton P: Effect of a high-protein, high-monounsaturated fat weight low carbohydrate diet on glycemic control and lipid levels in type 2 diabetes. Diabetes Care 25:425–430, 2002.

154. Parulkar AA, Pendergrass ML, Granda-Ayala R, et al: Nonhypoglycemic effects of thiazolidinediones. Ann Intern Med 134:61–71, 2001.

155. Parving HH, Chaturvedi N, Viberti GC, et al: Does microalbuminuria predict diabetic nephropathy? Diabetes 25:406–407, 2002.

156. Parving HH, Lehnert H, Brochner-Mortensen J, et al: The effect of irbesartan on the development of diabetic nephropathy in patients with type 2 diabetes. N Engl J Med 345:870–878, 2001.

157. Pavia C, Ferrer I, Valls C, et al: Total homocysteine in patients with type 1 diabetes. Diabetes Care 23:84–87, 2000.

158. Pepys MB: The acute phase response and C-reactive protein. In Weatherall DJ, Ledingham JGG, Warrell DA, (eds): Oxford Textbook of Medicines. New York, Oxford University Press, 1996, pp 1527–1533.

159. Pradhan AD, Manson JE, Rifai N, et al: C-reactive protein, interleukin 6, and risk of developing type 2 diabetes mellitus. JAMA 286:327–334, 2001.

160. Raskin P, Dole JF, Rappaport EB: Rosiglitazone improves glucose control in poorly controlled, insulin treated patients with type 2 diabetes mellitus [abstract]. Diabetes 48(suppl 1):A95–0404, 1999.

161. Ratner RE, Hirsch IB, Neifing JL, et al: Less hypoglycemia with insulin glargine in intensive insulin therapy for type 1 diabetes. U.S. Study Group of Insulin Glargine in Type 1 Diabetes. Diabetes Care 23:639–643, 2000.

162. Ravid M, Lang R, Rachmani R, et al: Long-term renoprotective effect of angiotensin-converting enzyme inhibition in non-insulin-dependent diabetes mellitus. A 7-year follow-up study. Arch Intern Med 156:286–289, 1996.

163. Reaven GM: Role of insulin resistance in human disease. Diabetes 37:1595–1607, 1988.

164. Report of the National Cholesterol Education Program Expert Panel on Detection, Evaluation, and Treatment of High Blood Cholesterol in Adults. The Exper Panel. Arch Intern Med 148:36–39, 1988.

165. Riddle MC: Evening insulin strategy. Diabetes Care 13:676–681, 1990.

166. Riddle MC, Hart J, Bingham P, et al: Combined therapy for obese type 2 diabetes: suppertime mixed insulin with daytime sulfonylurea. Am J Med Sci 303:151–156, 1992.

167. Riddle MC, Hart JS, Bouma DJ, et al: Efficacy of bedtime NPH insulin with daytime sulfonylurea for subpopulation of type 2 diabetes subjects. Diabetes Care 12:623–629, 1989.

168. Ridker PM, Cushman M, Stampfer MJ, et al: Inflammation, aspirin, and the risk of cardiovascular disease in apparently healthy men. N Engl J Med 336:973–979, 1997.

169. Ridker PM, Hennekens CH, Buring JE, et al: C-reactive protein and other markers of inflammation in the prediction of cardiovascular disease in women. N Engl J Med. 342:836–843, 2000.

170. Ridker PM, Rifai N, Pfeffer MA, et al: Long-term effects of pravastatin on plasma concentration of C-reactive protein: the Cholesterol and Recurrent Events (CARE) Investigators. Circulation 100:230–235, 1999.
171. Robins SJ, Collins D, Wittes JT, et al: Relation of gemfibrozil treatment and lipid levels with major coronary events: VA-HIT: A randomized controlled trial. JAMA 285:1585–1591, 2001.
172. Rolka DB, Fagot-Campagna A, Narayan KM: Aspirin use among adults with diabetes: Estimates from the Third National Health and Nutrition Examination Survey. Diabetes Care 24:197–201, 2001.
173. Rosenblatt S, Miskin B, Glazer NB, et al: The impact of pioglitazone on glycemic control and atherogenic dyslipidemia in patients with type 2 diabetes mellitus. Coron Artery Dis 12:413–423, 2001.
174. Rosenson RS, Tangney CC: Antiatherothrombotic properties of statins. Implications for cardiovascular event reduction. JAMA 279:1643–1650, 1998.
175. Rosenstock J, Schwartz, SL, Clark, CM, et al: Basal insulin therapy in type 2 diabetes. Diabetes Care 24:631–636, 2001.
176. Ross R. Atherosclerosis—an inflammatory disease. N Engl J Med 340:115–126, 1999.
177. Rossing K, Christensen PK, Jensen BR, et al: Dual blockade of the renin-angiotensin system in diabetic nephropathy. A randomized double-blind crossover study. Diabetes Care 25:95–100, 2002.
178. Rubin C, Egan J, Schneider R, et al: Combination therapy with pioglitazone and insulin in patients with type 2 diabetes. Diabetes 48(suppl 1):A110–474, 1999.
179. Rubins HB, Robins SJ, Collins D, et al. The Veterans Affairs high-density lipoprotein intervention trial: baseline characteristics of normocholesterolemic men with coronary artery disease and low levels of high-density lipoprotein cholesterol. Am J Cardiol 78:572–575, 1996.
180. Rubins HB, Robins SJ, Collins D, et al: Gemfibrozil for the secondary prevention of coronary heart disease in men with low levels of high-density lipoprotein cholesterol. N Eng J Med 341:410–418, 1999.
181. Schmidt MI, Duncan BB, Watson RL, et al: A metabolic syndrome in whites and African-Americans: the Atherosclerosis Risk in Communities baseline study. Diabetes Care 19:414–418, 1996.
182. Schrier RW, Estacio RO: The effect of angiotensin-converting enzyme inhibitors on the progression of nondiabetic renal disease: A pooled analysis of individual-patient data from 11 randomized, controlled trials. Ann Intern Med 135:138–139, 2001.
183. Schrier RW, Estacio RO, Esler A, et al: Effects of aggressive blood pressure control in normotensive type 2 diabetic patients on albuminuria, retinopathy and strokes. Kidney Int 61:1086–1097, 2002.
184. Shepherd J, Cobbe SM, Ford I, et al, for the West of Scotland Coronary Prevention Study Group. Prevention of coronary heart disease with pravastatin in men with hypercholesterolemia. N Engl J Med 333:1301–1307, 1995.
185. Singer DE, Nathan DM, Anderson KM, et al: Association of HbA$_{1c}$ with prevalent cardiovascular disease in the original cohort of the Framingham Heart Study. Diabetes 41:202–208, 1992.
186. Skyler JS, Cefalu WT, Kourides IA, et al: Efficacy of inhaled human insulin in type 1 diabetes mellitus: a randomised proof-of-concept study. Lancet 357:331–335, 2001.
187. Solomon CG, Hu FB, Stampfer MJ, et al: Moderate alcohol consumption and risk of coronary heart disease among women with type 2 diabetes mellitus. Circulation 102:494–499, 2000.

88. Stamler J, Vaccaro O, Neaton JD, et al: Diabetes, other risk factors, and 12-yr cardiovascular mortality for men screened in the multiple risk factor intervention trial. Diabetes Care 16:434–444, 1993.

89. Steering Committee of the Physicians' Health Study Research Group: Final report on the aspirin component of the ongoing Physicians' Health Study. N Engl J Med 321:129–135, 1989.

90. Steiner G. Diabetes Atherosclerosis Intervention Study (DAIS): a study conducted in cooperation with the World Health Organization. Diabetologia 39:1655–1661, 1996.

91. Stiko-Rahm A, Wiman B, Hamsten A, et al: Secretion of plasminogen activator inhibitor 1 from cultured human umbilical vein endothelial cells is induced by very-low-density lipoprotein. Arteriosclerosis 10:1067–1973, 1990.

92. Stratton IM, Adler AI, Andrew H, et al: Association of glycaemia with macrovascular and microvascular complications of type 2 diabetes (UKPDS 35): Prospective observational study. BMJ 321:405–412, 2000.

93. Tabaei BP, Al Kassab AS, Ilag LL, et al: Does microalbuminuria predict diabetic nephropathy? Diabetes Care 24:1560–1566, 2001.

94. The ETDRS Investigators: Aspirin effects on mortality and morbidity in patients with diabetes mellitus. JAMA 268:1292, 1992

95. The EUCLID Study Group: Randomised placebo-controlled trial of lisinopril in normotensive patients with insulin-dependent diabetes and normoalbuminuria or microalbuminuria. Lancet 349:1787–1792, 1997.

96. The Heart Outcomes Prevention Evaluation Study Investigators: Effects of an angiotensin-converting-enzyme inhibitor, ramipril, on cardiovascular events in high-risk patients. N Engl J Med 342:145–153, 2000.

97. The Hope Study Investigators. The HOPE (Heart Outcomes Prevention Evaluation) Study: The design of a large, simple randomized trial of an angiotensin-converting enzyme inhibitor (ramipril) and vitamin E in patients at high risk of cardiovascular events. Can J Cardiol 12:127–137, 1996.

98. The Scandinavian Simvastatin Survival Study Group: Randomised trial of cholesterol lowering in 4444 patients with coronary heart disease: the Scandinavian Simvastatin Survival Study (4S). Lancet 344:1383–1389, 1994.

99. TIMAD Study Group: Ticlopidine treatment reduces the progression of nonproliferative diabetic retinopathy. Arch Ophthalmol 108:1577–1583, 1990.

100. Tuomilehto J, Rastenyte D, Birkenhager WH, et al: Effects of calcium-channel blockade in older patients with diabetes and systolic hypertension. N Engl J Med 340:677–684, 1999.

101. Turner RC, Cull CA, Frighi V, et al: Glycemic control with diet, sulfonylurea, metformin, or insulin in patients with type 2 diabetes mellitus: Progressive requirement for multiple therapies (UKPDS 49). JAMA 281:2005–2012, 1999.

102. UK Prospective Diabetes Study Group: Cost effectiveness analysis of improved blood pressure control in hypertensive patients with type 2 diabetes: (UKPDS 40) BMJ 317:720–726, 1998.

103. UK Prospective Diabetes Study Group: Effect of intensive blood glucose control with metformin on complications in overweight patients with type 2 diabetes (UKPDS 34). Lancet 352:854–865, 1998.

104. UK Prospective Diabetes Study Group. Efficacy of atenolol and captopril in reducing risk of macrovascular and microvascular complications in type 2 diabetes: (UKPDS 39) BMJ 317:713–720, 1998.

105. UK Prospective Diabetes Study (UKPDS) Group: Intensive blood-glucose control with sulphonylureas or insulin compared with conventional treatment and risk of complications in patients with type 2 diabetes (UKPDS 33). Lancet 352:837–853, 1998.

206. UK Prospective Diabetes Study Group. Tight blood pressure control and risk of macrovascular and microvascular complications in type 2 diabetes: (UKPDS 38) BMJ 317:703–713, 1998.
207. Valmadrid CT, Klein R, Moss SE, et al: Alcohol intake and the risk of coronary heart disease mortality in persons with older-onset diabetes mellitus. JAMA 282:239–246, 1999.
208. Van Den Berghe G, Wouters P, Weekers F, et al: Intensive insulin therapy in critically ill patients. N Engl J Med 345:1359–1367, 2001.
209. Vasan RS, Larson MG, Leip EP, et al: Impact of high-normal blood pressure on the risk of cardiovascular disease. N Engl J Med 345:1291–1297, 2001.
210. Vaughan DE: Fibrinolytic balance, the renin-angiotensin system and atherosclerotic disease. Eur Heart J 19(suppl G):G9–G12, 1998.
211. Vegt FD, Dekker JM, Ruhé HG, et al: Hyperglycaemia is associated with all-cause and cardiovascular mortality in the Hoorn population: the Hoorn Study. Diabetologia 42:926–931, 1999.
212. Wald NJ, Watt HC, Law MR, et al: Homocysteine and ischemic heart disease. Results of a prospective study with implications regarding prevention. An Intern Med 158:862–867, 1998.
213. Watkins PB, Whitcomb RW: Hepatic dysfunction associated with troglitazone. N Engl J Med 338–916–917, 1998.
214. Wollesen F, Brattstrom L, Refsum H, et al: Plasma total homocysteine and cysteine in relation to glomerular filtration rate in diabetes mellitus. Kidney Int 55:1028–1035, 1999.
215. Wright A, Burden ACF, Paisey RB, et al. Sulfonylurea inadequacy. Efficacy of addition of insulin over 6 years in patients with type 2 diabetes in the U.K. Prospective Diabetes Study (UKPDS 57). Diabetes Care 25:330–336, 2002.
216. Yale JF, Valiquett TR, Ghazzi MN, et al: The effect of a thiazolidinedione drug, troglitazone, on glycemia in patients with type 2 diabetes mellitus poorly controlled with sulfonylurea and metformin: a multicenter, randomized, double-blind, placebo-controlled trial. Ann Intern Med 134:737–745, 2001.
217. Yamasaki Y Kawamori R, Matsushima H, et al: Asymptomatic hyperglycaemia is associated with increased intimal plus medial thickness of the carotid artery. Diabetologia 38:585–591, 1995.
218. Yki-Jarvinen H, Ryysy L, Nikkila K, et al: Comparison of bedtime insulin regimens in patients with type 2 diabetes mellitus: A randomized, controlled trial Ann Intern Med 130:389–396, 1999.
219. Yki-Jarvinen H, Dressler A, Ziemen M, et al: Less nocturnal hypoglycemia and better post dinner glucose control with bedtime insulin glargine compared with bedtime NPH insulin during combination therapy in type 2 diabetes. Diabetes Care 23:1130–1136, 2001.
220. Yu JG, Kruszynska YT, Mulford M, et al: A comparison of troglitazone and metformin on insulin requirements in euglycemic intensively insulin-treated type 2 diabetic patients. Diabetes 48:2414–2421, 1999.
221. Yudkin JS, Stehouwer CD, Emeis JJ, et al: C-reactive protein in healthy subjects: associations with obesity, insulin resistance, and endothelial dysfunction: a potential role for cytokines originating from adipose tissue: Arterioscler Thromb Vasc Biol. 19:972–978, 1999.
222. Zander M, Madsbad S, Madsen JL, Holst JJ: Effect of 6-week course of glucagon-like peptide 1 on glycaemic control, insulin sensitivity, and β-cell function in type 2 diabetes: a parallel-group study. Lancet 359:824–830, 2002.

25 Myths About Diabetes

chapter
11

1. *Split-dose (70/30) insulin before breakfast (two-thirds of total dose) and before supper is a good way to control blood glucose in type 1 diabetes.*

In type 1 diabetes, with little or no endogenous insulin secretion, the presupper NPH dose may cause hypoglycemia at 3–4 AM, particularly if the dosage is raised with intensive glycemic management. The proper time to give a PM dose of NPH is at bedtime in type 1 diabetes. In some patients bedtime NPH may peak early and cause nocturnal hypoglycemia. Insulin glargine helps alleviate such a problem. Regular or rapid-acting insulin should be given before each meal in intensive management programs.

2. *Standard urinary dipsticks for protein are good tools to screen for microalbuminuria.*

Standard urinary dipsticks for protein do not pick up amounts of urinary albumin in the microalbuminuria range (30–300 mg/24 hr). Special dipsticks that are sensitive in this range are available. However, laboratory measurement of a spot test (preferably overnight) or 24-hour specimen for albumin and creatinine is preferred for definitive diagnosis. It should be confirmed at least once. This point is important, for microalbuminuria may predict renal failure in type 1 diabetes and cardiovascular events in type 2 patients. ACE inhibitor or angiotensin receptor blocker therapy is indicated if microalbuminuria is found.

3. *Type 1 diabetes rarely has its onset after age 30.*

There are probably as many people with type 1 diabetes diagnosed over the age of 30 as there are under the age of 30. Older patients usually are thin and require insulin for glycemic control. Fasting C-peptide levels are usually below 0.6 ng/ml.

4. *People with type 1 diabetes eventually lose all pancreatic insulin secretory ability.*

Complete loss of insulin secretory function may not always be the case in type 1 diabetes. In particular, some beta-cell reserve may be present

197

at the time of diagnosis. Some evidence indicates that minimal insulin secretion may be retained by using intensive glycemic management with insulin from the time of diagnosis, particularly in older-onset (over age 20) type 1 patients. In addition, African Americans may present with ketoacidosis, yet may retain beta-cell function after insulin treatment.

5. *Increased urinary albumin excretion is an inevitable consequence of type 1 diabetes.*

About 30–40% of people with type 1 diabetes have increased urinary protein excretion. This incidence appears to be decreasing, presumably because of more intensive glucose and early blood pressure control. Prevention of microalbuminuria by early ACE inhibitor or ARB therapy is under study.

6. *People with type 1 diabetes often have an atherogenic lipid profile and/or hypertension.*

Uncomplicated patients with type 1 diabetes who are well managed on insulin usually have normal lipid/lipoprotein levels and are nor-motensive (BP < 130/80 mmHg). If albuminuria occurs, an atherogenic profile (high cholesterol, LDL-C, triglycerides, low HDL-C) is often present. Blood pressure often rises above 130/80 mmHg, and cardiovascular risk is magnified greatly.

7. *Below the threshold value of HbA1c, there is little or no risk of retinopathy and/or nephropathy progression.*

The DCCT explored this issue in detail in type 1 diabetes and found no evidence of a threshold value of HbA1c for retinopathy or nephropathy. The UKPDS found similar results in newly discovered type 2 patients.

8. *A type 1 diabetic patient who has frequent episodes of hypo-glycemia is a good candidate for insulin pump therapy.*

This is not always the case. Candidates for insulin pump therapy must be carefully screened before starting such therapy. A prospective pump user must demonstrate adherence to a regimen of frequent (at least 4 times/day) blood glucose monitoring as well as evidence of choosing appropriate basal and premeal insulin dose according to a plan defined by the patient and the health care team. Pump therapy may reduce the risk of severe hypoglycemia only in patients who understand and adhere to a mutually developed treatment plan.

9. *It is critical to achieve a HbA1c goal of less than 7% to prevent pro-gression of retinopathy.*

Although a HbA1c level of < 7% is a goal of therapy based on DCCT and UKPDS results, it is often impossible to achieve and maintain this degree of glycemic control in type 1 diabetes without the risk of severe hypoglycemia. This was also a limiting factor in type 2 diabetes in the UKPDS. If hypoglycemia that requires assistance from another person occurs, one must use a less intensive regimen. Fortunately, lowering of

HbA1c from any elevated level decreases the risk of progression of retinopathy.

10. *Because insulin pump therapy is expensive and technically challenging, its use is decreasing among people with type 1 diabetes.*

Insulin pump usage is increasing in type 1 diabetes. Partial or complete coverage by insurance companies for insulin pump therapy is usually obtained after physician justification. There are excellent teaching modules for insulin pump therapy, and many physicians and nurses have become experts in this discipline. Studies indicate that patient satisfaction is high and that severe hypoglycemia is decreased with insulin pump use. Some evidence also indicates that glycemic control is improved with pump therapy compared with multiple daily injections.

11. *Patients with type 2 diabetes and persistently elevated glucose and HbA1c levels would be well controlled if they simply complied with the exercise and meal plan.*

Although this may be true in a minority of patients, it is not the issue in most. Type 2 diabetes appears to have a natural history of progressive beta-cell failure from the time of first diagnosis, demonstrated by the United Kingdom Prospective Diabetes Study (UKPDS) in patients randomized to a diet and exercise program as well as those on sulfonylurea, metformin, or insulin therapy. Beta-cell failure probably plays a major role in the increased need for multiple pharmacologic therapy as the duration of type 2 diabetes increases.

12. *An overnight fast is required for accurate cholesterol levels.*

Plasma cholesterol levels are not acutely affected by a meal. However, plasma triglyceride levels may rise after eating, and there may be a slight decrease in plasma HDL-C concentration. For this reason, an overnight fast of at least 8 hours is recommended before measuring a complete plasma lipid profile.

13. *Hypertriglyceridemia is not a cardiovascular risk factor for people with diabetes.*

Studies have shown that an elevated plasma triglyceride level is a risk factor for coronary heart disease in people with diabetes. Furthermore, lowering of plasma triglyceride and raising plasma HDL-C levels with fibrate therapy reduces cardiovascular risk in type 2 diabetes. Many investigators believe that postprandial hypertriglyceridemia is a major contributor to this cardiovascular risk.

14. *Good evidence indicates that intensive glycemic control delays the progression of atherosclerotic vascular disease in type 2 diabetes.*

Although progression of microvascular disease of eyes and kidneys may be delayed by intensive glucose management, no prospective studies demonstrate that this principle applies to macrovascular disease. There was optimism that the UKPDS would give such information, but results were not significant. The NIH and the VA system have ongoing large-scale, prospective, randomized trials that address this important issue.

15. *Type 2 diabetes rarely has its onset before age 30.*

Obese, insulin-resistant type 2 patients under the age of 30 are appearing with increased frequency. Occasionally they may be members of families with a strong heredity predisposition for diabetes (i.e., maturity onset diabetes of youth (MODY). More frequently, they are found in people of American Indian, Hispanic, or African American descent. Onset typically occurs during puberty and has been related to excessive growth hormone secretion. Acanthosis nigricans and/or polycystic ovary syndrome may be present; both are useful clinical clues. In a recent report, 24% of obese children (aged 4–10) who were referred to an academic obesity clinic had impaired glucose tolerance.

16. *People with type 2 diabetes rarely have an atherogenic lipid profile.*

At least 30–40% of people with type 2 diabetes in the U.S. have lipid or lipoprotein values that promote progression of atherosclerosis. Classically, there is an elevated plasma level of triglycerides and small, dense LDL molecules as well as a low plasma HDL-C level.

17. *Microalbuminuria is a predictor of eventual renal insufficiency in type 2 diabetes.*

Microalbuminuria predicts cardiovascular death in type 2 diabetes. This relationship is magnified by persistently elevated HbA1c levels. It is also a predictor of renal insufficiency in type 2 diabetes. Recent prospective trials of ARB therapy in type 2 diabetic patients with hypertension and albuminuria showed that the rate of progression of renal insufficiency is decreased by ARB therapy.

18. *Glucose elevation is not a predictor of coronary heart disease.*

Many studies have identified elevated HbA1c or fasting or postprandial glucose levels as independent predictors of coronary heart disease. This finding suggests that intensive glycemic control could reduce the risk for cardiovascular disease. However, no long-term intervention trials have determined whether intensive glucose control alters the course of coronary heart disease (or other cardiovascular events) in diabetes. The UKPDS showed a nonsignificant trend toward reducing the risk of myocardial infarction in type 2 patients with a policy of intensive glycemic control.

19. *Exogenous insulin administration produces hyperinsulinemia and has been shown to increase the risk for cardiovascular disease in diabetes.*

Although some epidemiologic evidence supports the view that endogenous hyperinsulinemia may predict coronary heart disease in nondiabetic males, no prospective trial data support the view that exogenous insulin increases coronary events in people with type 1 or type 2 diabetes. In the UKPDS, the DCCT, and the University Group Diabetes

Program. (UGDP), intensive insulin therapy was not associated with an increase in cardiovascular events.

20. *Elevated HbA1c, altered lipid profiles, and hypertension explain the increased cardiovascular risk seen in type 2 diabetes.*

Although it is likely that these three indicators play major roles, recent work has defined less traditional cardiovascular risk markers in people with diabetes. One of these is c-reactive protein (CRP), as determined by a highly sensitive assay. CRP is a marker of vascular inflammation. Another is fibrinogen; elevated levels, which are commonly seen in poorly controlled diabetes, are predictive of heart attacks. Plasma levels of plasminogen activator inhibitor (PAI-1), an inhibitor of clot lysis, may be predictive, as may plasma homocysteine levels. As this list becomes complete and prospective trials are done, we will have many logical targets for preventive therapy.

21. *Aspirin's effect to lower the risk for myocardial infarction in type 2 diabetes is mediated solely through its inhibition of platelet cyclooxygenase and, therefore, thromboxane synthesis.*

Although this is a major mechanism of aspirin's action, other results of aspirin therapy may play a role in reducing the risk of vascular thrombosis. In the Physician's Health Study, CRP was a predictor of coronary events, and aspirin therapy was particularly effective in preventing events in CRP-positive people, probably via its anti-inflammatory actions. Furthermore, platelet PAI-1 release has been shown to be stimulated by the thromboxane precursor, arachidonic acid. Aspirin in high doses blocks arachidonic acid stimulation of platelet PAI-1 release. This is another mechanism by which aspirin could influence coronary thrombosis.

22. *A fasting plasma glucose value of 120 mg/dl is of no consequence.*

Fasting plasma glucose values of 110–125 mg/dl represent impaired fasting glucose (IFG), which the ADA has defined as pre-diabetes. In particular, a high-risk person, such as an African or Hispanic American, will have a significant chance of being (or becoming) diabetic. A 75-gm oral glucose tolerance test should be done to evaluate the possibility of either diabetes (2 hour value > 200 mg/dl) or impaired glucose tolerance (2 hour value of 140–200 mg/dl). At the very least, a patient with FPG of 120 mg/dl should be followed with yearly fasting plasma glucose determinations and instructed about lifestyle issues, including regular exercise and weight control.

23. *The nonsteroidal anti-inflammatory drug (NSAID) ibuprofen, may be substituted for aspirin for prevention of vascular events in diabetes.*

Although some NSAIDs are weak inhibitors of platelet thromboxane release, in contrast to aspirin, the effect does not persist, even with daily dosing. Of clinical importance is the finding that 400 mg of ibuprofen, taken before aspirin (either in the morning or 3 times daily on the previous day), blocks aspirin's antithrombotic effect: inhibition of thromboxane production. Cyclooxygenase-2 (COX-2) inhibitors, acetaminophen, and diclofenac do not have that effect. If indicated for arthritis or other reasons, these drugs are preferable to use in combination with aspirin rather than ibuprofen if cardioprotection is the goal of aspirin therapy.

24. *All people with diabetes should be on ACE inhibitor therapy.*

This is an overstatement of the evidence from collaborative clinical trials. In type 1 diabetes, ACE inhibitor therapy is recommended only as a first-line agent for treatment of BP ≥ 130/80 mmHg and in patients with micro- or macroalbuminuria. The HOPE study showed that type 2 diabetics with high cardiovascular risk (hypertension, elevated total cholesterol level, low HDL cholesterol level, cigarette smoking, microalbuminuria, or clinical evidence of vascular disease) had a reduced risk for cardiovascular events when treated with the ACE inhibitor ramipril. Because some type 2 diabetic patients do not have high cardiovascular risk (as defined in HOPE), ACE inhibitor therapy should not be used in all people with type 2 diabetes.

25. *In patients with the dyslipidemia characteristic of type 2 diabetes (elevated fasting plasma triglycerides and low HDL cholesterol levels), a nutrition plan and an exercise program are usually effective in achieving the recommended goals of therapy.*

Although weight reduction, a diet high in monounsaturated fats, and an exercise program are beneficial in the treatment of diabetic dyslipidemia, they often do not result in normal plasma lipid levels. Furthermore, excellent glycemic control may not be associated with the recommended lipid goals, especially in the case of low HDL cholesterol levels. To achieve the goals of < 100 mg/dl (LDL-C), < 150 mg/dl (triglycerides), and > 45 mg/dl (HDL-C in men) or > 55 mg/dl (HDL-C in women), drugs that affect lipoprotein metabolism are often needed. The first target is LDL-C < 100 mg/dl, usually achieved easily with statin therapy. If the other goals are not met, the addition of a fibrate or niacin, with monitoring of liver and muscle enzymes, is indicated.

Type 2 Diabetes: Illustrative Cases

chapter

12

Early Treatment

Patient No. 1

A 52-year-old white man was self-referred because he thought that he had diabetes. His father, paternal grandfather, and four uncles have had type 2 diabetes. He borrowed his father's glucose monitoring device and checked his prebreakfast blood glucose on 5 successive days 2 months before he was seen. The average fasting blood glucose level was 158 mg/dl. He dieted and lost 7 pounds and now wished an opinion about the diagnosis and treatment of his suspected diabetes. The remainder of the history was noncontributory, except that he had a glucose tolerance test done about 6 years ago and was told it was at "the top of normal." He also complained of slight loss of erectile function.

Physical examination: height, 73 inches; weight, 236 lb; BMI, 31 kg/m^2; BP, 148/86 mmHg. Background retinopathy was present. Laboratory values: HbA1c, 7.1%; cholesterol, 213; triglycerides, 204; HDL-C, 43; LDL-C, 129 mg/dl. Spot urine albumin/creatinine ratio: 4 mg/gm. Fasting plasma insulin, 21μU/ml; C-peptide, 1.5 ng/ml; thyroid-stimulating hormone normal; EKG, normal.

The diagnosis of type 2 diabetes is confirmed by the HbA1c of 7.1%. He is obese, with a BMI of 31 kg/m^2. Blood pressure is above the ideal level of 130/80 mmHg, and he has elevated plasma triglycerides, normal HDL-C, and slightly elevated LDL-C levels. Thus, he may be viewed as a mild example of metabolic syndrome in view of obesity, dyslipidemia, and borderline hypertension. His cardiovascular risk is high. He agreed to follow a regular nutrition and exercise plan designed to lose weight and improve metabolic control. One year after he was first seen, he had lost 20 lb and HbA1c had fallen from 7.1% to 5.2%. His blood pressure was 110/80 mmHg. Lipid profile did not improve, however: cholesterol, 230; triglycerides, 160; HDL-C, 55; LDL-C, 143 mg/dl. He was started on atorvastatin, 5 mg/day; cholesterol fell to 200 and LDL-C to 105 mg/dl.

Over the next year he gained 12 lb., and HbA1c rose to 7.4%. Glucophage was started, 1 gm twice daily, and HbA1c dropped to 6.5% in 6 months.

This patient had three aspects of the metabolic syndrome. He responded to strict weight management with optimal glucose control but probably will need additional oral agents of a different class as time progresses. The dyslipidemia is fairly well managed on atorvastatin in low doses. It is likely that an increase to 10 mg in the future will be needed to reach target LDL-C goal of < 100 mg/dl. In view of high cardiovascular risk, he is maintained on enteric coated aspirin, 81mg/day. Blood pressure remains < 130/80 mmHg, and he has no microalbuminuria. ACE inhibitor therapy is a consideration because of his high cardiovascular risk, based on the results of the HOPE Study.

Patient No. 2

A 72-year-old white man was found to have diabetes a few weeks before he was first seen in October, 1999. He had previous fasting glucose values of 95 (1997) and 167 (1998) and was found to have a current value of 149 mg/dl (1999). Diagnosis of diabetes was confirmed by HbA1c of 7.1%. Fingerstick values ranged from 77–146 mg/dl (fasting) and as high as 121 after supper. He had a history of hypertension for several years, adequately managed by calcium channel blocker therapy. His history was otherwise noncontributory, except for a 20-lb weight gain in the past few years.

Physical examination: height, 73 inches; weight, 200 lb; BMI, 27 kg/m²; BP, 134/73 mmHg. Physical examination was otherwise completely negative.

The diabetes did not respond optimally to diet therapy. After glucophage was added, HbA1c became normal, and the patient lost 7 lb. His elevated LDL-C responded well to atorvastatin 10 mg/day, and HDL-C rose. Blood pressure was 148–155/70–75mmHg on calcium channel blocker therapy and fell to 132/59 mmHg when a low dose of ACE inhibitor was added.

Like the first patient, he had mild diabetes that eventually required

Physical and Serial Laboratory Values							
Date	Wt(lb)	HbA1c	Chol	TG	HDL-C	LDL-C	Therapy
10/99	200	7.1%	202	179	33	133	Diet
10/2000	202	7.4%	219	218	34	141	Atorvastatin, 10mg + Glucophage, 500 b.i.d.
4/2001	194	6.6%	148	84	42	89	
9/2001	195	6.0%					

oral agent therapy for optimal glucose control. Metformin was chosen in both cases because of the UKPDS data showing a reduction in the risk for cardiovascular events with metformin therapy (as opposed to sulfonylureas, insulin, or diet alone) in recently diagnosed type 2 diabetic patients. The dyslipidemia responded to atorvastatin therapy, diet, and exercise.

This patient had no microalbuminuria, but systolic hypertension was inadequately managed on calcium channel blocker therapy. BP control improved when an ACE inhibitor was added. In view of the cardioprotection afforded by ACE inhibitor therapy in type 2 diabetics with high cardiovascular risk (HOPE Study), this is the indicated therapy. As time progresses, he may well need the addition of other agents to his present regimen of blood glucose and BP control.

Medical Nutrition Therapy Followed By Single and Dual Oral Agent Therapy

Patient No. 3

A 50-year-old white man was first found to have fasting hyperglycemia in 1996 (154 mg/dl), and in 1997 the level was 152 mg/dl. He was first seen in June, 1997, and the diagnosis was confirmed by a HbA1c value of 7.2%. His father had type 2 diabetes. His medical history included a weight gain from about 200 lb (in college) to present weight of 276 lb. He had a history of intermittent hypertension, not treated.

Physical examination: weight, 276 lb; height, 72 inches; BMI, 37kg/m²; BP 146/82 mmHg; obese and ruddy-faced. Examination otherwise negative.

This patient is an excellent example of metabolic syndrome. He has centripetal obesity, with a 76-lb weight gain over about 25 years, hypertension, dyslipidemia, diabetes, and microalbuminuria. He had reasonably good glycemic control with a nutrition and exercise program but required metformin, 1.0 gm twice daily, until 1/01, when HbA1c rose to 8.6%. At that time, diet and exercise were reemphasized and glimeperide, 4 mg, was added, with a fall in HbA1c to 7.3%. This is compatible with the usual glycemic effect of these two agents in combination. However, unless he can successfully sustain weight reduction, he will progress to needing a third oral agent, probably a thiazolidinedione. Alternatively, bedtime glargine insulin may then be added. It is likely that insulin will be eventually needed to maintain HbA1c < 8%, with a goal of < 7%.

His cardiovascular risk is a serious medical problem. The hypertension is not well controlled by an ARB plus low-dose thiazide, and a beta

Physical and Serial Laboratory Values

Date	Wt(lb)	BP (mmHg)	HbA1c	Chol	TG	HDL-C	LDL-C	Urine mg Alb/24 hr	Homocysteine μMol/L	Therapy
6/97	276	146/82	7.2%	208	254	29	127			Diet, exercise ARB, HCTZ
8/97	271	144/84	6.1%							
10/97	273	150/100	6.4%	233	356	45	117	90		Atorvastatin
2/98	267	140/90	6.8%							
10/98	277	140/70	7.1%							Metformin
2/99	273	150/92	6.2%	194	308	51	81	115	12.9	
11/99	270	160/90	5.9%	214	223	55	114	117	14.5	
9/00	266	120/80	6.5%	187	202	52	95			
1/01	271	140/84	8.6%							Glimeperide added
11/01	275	165/87	7.3%	174	125	55	94		12.8	

blocker or calcium channel blocker will be added. The dyslipidemia has responded well to atorvastatin, 10 mg/day. Optimally, the microalbuminuria should drop about 50% or more, and this decrease may be seen with improved BP control. One option is to add an ACE inhibitor to present therapy. Finally, he has elevated plasma homocysteine levels (over 12), as do many type 2 diabetic patients with metabolic syndrome and albuminuria. This problem is presently being managed with increasing doses of folic acid, and he is maintained on low-dose aspirin therapy.

We have had some success in patients of this type by referral to an intensive weight management center, where a very low calorie approach, followed by a high-protein, low-carbohydrate, low-fat hypocaloric meal plan is instituted. He has been counseled to explore this program, and we have enlisted his wife's support. In any case, it is clear that an intensive multifactorial approach is clearly needed in this "mild diabetic."

Patient No. 4

A 60-year-old oral surgeon was first seen in September, 1995, after the recent discovery of diabetes mellitus. He gave a history of a random blood glucose of 205 mg/dl 5 years previously, and a fasting value of 110 mg/dl about 2 years ago. In July, 1995, fasting plasma glucose was 201 mg/dl; in August, it was 254 mg/dl; and in September, it was 268 mg/dl. He had nocturia (× 2), no thirst or polyuria. Weight had been constant at 165–170 lb for many years. He had a history of hypertension, treated with a calcium channel blocker. Other medical history was noncontributory.

Physical examination: height, 69 inches; weight, 167 lb; BMI 25kg/m²; BP 160/88 mmHg. Examination was otherwise normal.

The HbA1c responded well to a nutrition plan and a combination of metformin, 1.0 gm twice daily, plus glipizide (XL), 10 mg/day. However, he developed persistent bigeminy, with some correlation of premature ventricular contractions and low fingerstick glucose values plus symptoms of hypoglycemia. The sulfonylurea was stopped (8/96), and he was maintained on metformin alone. However, in 6/97, metformin was stopped because of GI complaints. Troglitazone was started (11/97) and changed to pioglitazone when troglitazone was removed from the market. Over this period, HbA1c values stayed in an excellent range, but his weight increased from 173 to 192 lb. He has no symptoms or findings of congestive heart failure and has unilateral edema due to deep vein thrombosis on the left.

His cardiovascular risk profile has been on target with a combination of ACE inhibitor, calcium channel blocker, and a beta blocker for hypertension and atorvastatin, 10 mg for dyslipidemia. He has developed microalbuminuria.

Physical and Serial Laboratory Values

Date	Wt(lb)	BP (mmHg)	HbA1c	Chol	TG	HDL-C	LDL-C	Urine mg Alb/24 hr	Therapy
9/95	167	160/88	8.8%	177	210	30	105	<30	Metformin, glipizide, ACE-I, Ca Ch + β blocker
8/96	174	128/78	6.4%						
8/97	173	160/80	5.9%	173	212	25	106	13	D/C glipizide(hypoglycemia)
12/98	180	150/80	6.1%	172	205	26	105		D/C metformin(GI)
1/1000	186	130/70	6.9%	134	197	27	68	19	Pioglitazone, Atorvastatin
11/1000	193	146/78	5.7%	126	123	40	61	35	
8/1001	192	136/80	5.4%	123	140	38	57	43	

This patient illustrates potential hazards of dual therapy with metformin and a sulfonylurea. He developed recurrent arrhythmias, which were well documented by EKGs, and occurred in the late mornings when he also had symptomatic hypoglycemia along with low fingerstick BG readings. This problem has disappeared since switching to thiazolidinedione therapy and adding a cardiospecific beta blocker to his antihypertensive therapy. This is a rare example of a potentially dangerous arrhythmia demonstrated by EKG concomitant with symptomatic hypoglycemia, which was confirmed by fingerstick testing. One can only speculate about the possible influence of sulfonylurea therapy and hypoglycemia in this clinical setting. The patient's course also illustrates the problems of weight gain in people who respond to thiazolidinedione therapy. The 19-lb. weight gain is the major challenge now, and that risk must be balanced against the perceived benefits of thiazolidinedione therapy. He is monitored for the development of congestive heart failure. Long-term experience and clinical trials with these new agents are needed to give a clear perspective about these issues.

Therapy With Three or Four Oral Agents with or without Insulin

Patient No. 5

A 54-year-old white woman was first seen in July, 1998, after moving from the United Kingdom to the United States. About 2 years previously, she developed polyuria, polydipsia, a groin abscess, and a 40-lb weight loss over 1 year. Diabetes was diagnosed, and she was placed on a diet and 5 mg of glyburide daily. Metformin, 850 mg twice daily, was added after about 3 months of glyburide monotherapy. She had a daughter, now 23 years old, who weighed 9 lb 12 oz and required a caesarean operation. Blood glucose was not checked during the pregnancy. She had a grandmother and an aunt with type 2 diabetes. Both parents died of coronary artery disease in their 50s. There was a 10 year history of hypertension, treated with atenolol, 50 mg/day. She also had a history of hyperlipidemia, treated with simvastatin, 10 mg daily. She was menopausal, treated with an estrogen/progestin combination.

Physical examination: height, 66 inches; weight, 182 lb; BP, 170/82 mmHg. Centripetal obesity. Fundi negative except for increased A/V ratio. No abnormalities of heart, lungs, breasts, or abdomen. Pulses palpable, no edema, neurologic examination negative.

The diagnosis of type 2 diabetes was confirmed by repeated C-peptide values from 3.2 to 4.5 mg/ml. She had many characteristics of the metabolic syndrome: centripetal obesity, BMI 33kg/m^2 after therapy, hyper-

Physical and Serial Laboratory Values

Date	Wt(lb)	BP (mmHg)	HbA1c	Chol	TG	HDL-C	LDL-C	Urine mgAlb/24 hr	Therapy
7/98	182	170/82	9.8%	315	410	37	178	28	3 oral agents
11/98	187	130/80	8.0%	216	192	43	135		ACE-I, atenolol atorvastatin 40mg
4/99	200	120/60	7.4%	203	254	31	121	21	
11/99	204	130/80	7.7%	208	175	40	133		4 oral agents
10/2000	206	120/60	6.8%	182	148	38	114	24	
7/2001	207	108/68	6.9%	212	186	46	129	30	

tension, and dyslipidemia. She may have had gestational diabetes 23 years before we saw her in view of the history of a large infant. Her strong family history of coronary artery disease plus metabolic syndrome placed her at high risk for a myocardial infarction. She had no retinopathy or microalbuminuria. To achieve HbA1c goal of < 7%, she required therapy with four oral agents: a sulfonylurea, metformin, a thiazolidinedione, and a meglitinide. Lipid profile improved but did not reach target with high doses of atorvastatin, good glycemic control, and counseling about nutrition and exercise. She was well managed on atenolol plus ACE inhibitor for hypertension and also took enteric-coated aspirin, 81 mg/day. Postmenopausal hormone therapy was continued since she has not had a myocardial infarction, and its possible cardioprotective action is considered to outweigh its probable contribution to weight gain and dyslipidemia.

It is likely that this patient will require insulin therapy soon. The long-term effects of four different oral agents are unknown and such therapy is expensive. Addition of a bedtime dosage of glargine insulin to produce FBG of 80–120 mg/dl should allow the use of a combination of insulin and one or two oral agents (ie., thiazolidinedione and metformin). The dyslipidemia may be improved by increasing her atorvastatin dose to 80 mg in order to get LDL-C below 100 mg/dl. Addition of nicotinic acid is an option, but it would complicate glycemic control by increasing insulin resistance. Medical nutrition therapy and a regular walking program continue to be encouraged.

This patient illustrates that aggressive multifactorial cardioprotective therapy is usually indicated and difficult to accomplish perfectly, particularly in a patient with metabolic syndrome and longstanding poorly controlled type 2 diabetes.

Patient No. 6

A 70-year-old white woman was first seen in April, 1998, when random blood glucose values by fingersticks were 285 and 273 mg/dl. About 6 years before her first visit, her primary care physician told her she had a "tendency towards diabetes" and should go on a diet. At the age of 50 she weighed 130 lb; her present weight was 185 lb. Her father had type 2 diabetes. She had three children, 48–50 years ago, with no knowledge of diabetes during pregnancy; all three infants weighed less than 8 lb at birth.

Physical examination: height, 67 inches; weight, 185 lb; BP, 140/86 mmHg. Except for obesity, the examination was normal.

This patient probably had type 2 diabetes for at least 6 years before she was first seen—a common issue in type 2 diabetes. Early recognition with intensive management of risk factors is critical for successful

Physical and Serial Laboratory Values

Date	Wt(lb)	BP (mmHg)	HbA1c	Chol	TG	HDL-C	LDL-C	Urine mgAlb/24 hr	Therapy
4/98	185	140/86	11.4%	316	335	47	202	45	2 orals ACE-I Atorvastatin, 10mg
7/98	190	120/70	8.3%	202	245	55	98		3 orals
2/99	190	160/88	7.2%	184	252	51	83	15	
8/99	190	150/82	7.1%						
2/00	193	126/76	6.7%	210	248	53	108	15	c-peptide 1.0mg/ml
8/00	185	130/80	8.0%	205	209	52	111		Add glargine hs
3/01	190	151/82	8.1%						Ca channel blocker
9/01	188	172/87	7.8%					Spot	
3/02	190	152/83	6.4%					20mg/gm Cr.	

long-term care. When first seen, the patient had a seriously atherogenic lipid profile and uncontrolled diabetes. She appeared to respond to triple oral therapy for the hyperglycemia: metformin, sulfonylurea (or a meglitinide), and a thiazolidinedione. She had borderline elevation of hepatic enzymes that never reached the stop point of three times the upper limit of normal. Despite triple oral agent therapy, she progressed to insulin therapy; pancreatic beta-cell deficiency was documented by a low fasting C-peptide level. The present approach to intensive glycemic therapy is bedtime glargine insulin to produce FBG in the range of 80–110 mg/dl and daytime combination of metformin and a thiazolidinedione. This regimen has successfully reduced HbA1c to <7%.

Her other problems are suboptimal management of blood pressure and lipids. As is usually the case, she requires more than one antihypertensive agent for BP control. The slightly elevated LDL-C level should fall below 100 mg/dl with higher statin doses. She takes 81 mg of enteric-coated aspirin daily and works to keep her weight down by walking and watching caloric intake. Urinary microalbuminuria has been intermittently present and should be controlled by BP and glycemic control.

Treatment of Type 2 Diabetic Patients With Complications

Patient No. 7

A 70-year-old white man was first seen in February, 1999. He gave a history of type 2 diabetes for 32 years, treated with one oral agent daily. His present therapy was glipizide (XL), 10 mg/day. His major complaints were impotence for many years, progressive leg weakness, shooting pains down both legs, progressive loss of sensation in his feet, and burning of the soles of the feet. Gait had become wobbly, and he had difficulty maintaining balance, with one episode of falling. He had a past history of coronary artery bypass in 1985. Hypertension was diagnosed, and his most recent therapy was an ARB for about 2 years. Cholesterol had been elevated and treated with simvastatin, 20 mg/day. He had lost weight from 300 to 231 lb over the past few years.

Physical examination: weight, 231 lb; height 78 inches; BP, 160/90 mmHg. The patient walked unsteadily with a cane. Other findings included background diabetic retinopathy, midline sternotomy scar, absent light touch from below knees to soles of feet, loss of vibratory sense over malleoli and great toes, absent ankle jerks, extensor weakness of thighs with loss of muscle mass, and palpable peripheral pulses with no edema.

Physical and Serial Laboratory Values

Date	Wt(lb)	BP (mmHg)	HbA1c	Chol	TG	HDL-C	LDL-C	Urine mgAlb/24 hr	Misc. Rx
2/99	231	160/90	11%	208	464	26	—	64	Triple orals Atorvastatin 10mg
8/99	247	150/90	8.3%	171	329	28	77		ARB + HCTZ
12/99	257	160/98	7.8%						Insulin Ca Channel Blocker
2/00	264	126/80	7.0%	160	200	35	85		
8/00	260	140/60	7.8%						
3/01	264	160/82	7.5%						

The patient's major complaint was progressive diabetic neuropathy. He had the findings of amyotrophic diabetes with severe peripheral sensory and autonomic neuropathy. This problem responded well to a regimen of more intensive glycemic control with metformin, a sulfonylurea, and a thiazolidinedione. However, glycemic control was not optimal, and insulin was added. He has required large doses (over 100 U) in addition to thiazolidione and metformin therapy and will need further adjustment when next seen. Blood pressure control has required an ARB, thiazide, and calcium channel blocker. A cardiospecific beta blocker may be added, since pulse rate is over 70 beats/min. Lipids have responded well to statin therapy, except for persistently low HDL-C. Fibrates should be added in view of his past CABG and high cardiovascular risk. He takes 81 mg of enteric-coated aspirin.

Because of his microalbuminuria and coronary artery disease, plasma homocysteine levels were checked and found to be elevated (17 μMol/L; normal range: 4–12). Because of this finding and his high cardiovascular risk, he was placed on folic acid, 2 mg/day, with a resultant fall in homocysteine level to 12 μMol/L. Higher doses of folic acid and 50 mg of vitamin B_6 and 1000 μg of B_{12} will be added to achieve a lower plasma level of homocysteine and to avoid neuropathy progression.

He has seen dramatic improvement in strength, gait, unsteadiness, and general well-being. The impotence and peripheral sensory neuropathy have not changed except that the burning of the soles of the feet has disappeared. He continues with a physical therapy and an exercise program to regain muscle strength and to help with weight control. Intensive glycemic management with insulin, a nutritional program, vitamins, and exercise conditioning are necessary for return of some function in this type of diabetic neuropathy.

Patient No. 8

A 60-year-old white man was first seen in December, 1999. He had a 2-year history of type 2 diabetes and was placed on metformin and a sulfonylurea with good blood glucose response. He had a history of 3 packs per day of cigarette smoking, which he stopped 14 years ago. He had always been heavy, with a maximal weight of 275 lb after stopping smoking. He lost to 230 lb before diabetes was found and then regained to 248 lb. He had diabetic retinopathy, with laser therapy planned, and also was aware that his cholesterol and blood pressure had been elevated in the past.

Physical examination: weight, 298 lb; height, 69 inches; BP, 160/80 mmHg. Bilateral preproliferative retinopathy, heart, lungs; abdomen negative except for centripetal obesity; weak dorsalis pedis and posterial tibial pulses; absent ankle jerks; no edema.

Serial Physical and Laboratory Values

Date	Wt(lb)	BP (mmHg)	HbA1c	Chol	TG	HDL-C	LDL-C	Urine mgAlb/24 hr	Therapy
12/99	248	160/80	7.1%	246	442	44	—	198	Metformin, sulf. ACE-I, statin,
4/00	244	140/78	6.8%	169	370	49	41	199	Laser Rx
7/00	237	140/80	5.5%						CABG 7/00
11/00	228	126/88	5.5%	176	253	46	79	186	ARB(cough)
6/01	236	119/63	6.8%						
9/01	238	122/65	ô.4%	180	200	50	90		

Glycemic regulation has been excellent, and he is most recently managed on metformin alone. Despite weight control, exercise, lipid and blood pressure management, and low-dose aspirin therapy, he developed angina while swimming and was found to need a triple coronary artery bypass in July, 2000. He had the components of metabolic syndrome, with centripetal obesity, hypertension, dyslipidemia, and microalbuminuria. Intensive cardiovascular risk reduction measures will continue.

He also has the microvascular complications of retinopathy, which required laser therapy, and microalbuminuria. He developed cough on ACE inhibitor therapy, and BP has responded well to ARB plus HCTZ. This regimen, plus excellent diabetic control, should keep the microvascular disease of the kidney and retina from progressing. He has normal plasma homocysteine levels and normal renal and thyroid function. He has a high fasting C-peptide level of 6.5 ng/ml, which suggests insulin resistance. He should continue to do well on insulin sensitizer therapy, diet, and exercise.

Summary of Intensive Management

chapter
13

Type 1 Diabetes

Pathophysiology

Autoimmune destruction of the beta cells of the pancreas is the primary cause of type 1 diabetes. Loss of beta-cell function may also occur by nonautoimmune mechanisms. In either case, insulin therapy is needed for life and usually is required at the time of diagnosis or shortly thereafter. If intensive glycemic management with insulin is successfully instituted from the time of first recognition of type 1 diabetes, a minimal amount of beta-cell function may be preserved. Intensive glycemic regulation is easier in such patients than in patients with complete beta cell loss, and the progression of microvascular complications is delayed.

Intensive Glycemic Management

The Diabetes Control and Complications Trial (DCCT) demonstrated that intensive glycemic management of people with uncomplicated diabetes mellitus by a team approach significantly reduces progression of diabetic retinopathy, urinary albumin excretion (an index of nephropathy), and clinical evidence of peripheral sensory and autonomic neuropathy. Intensive glycemic management is mandatory in pregnancy to ensure normal outcomes.

Because insulin deficiency is virtually absolute in type 1 diabetes, insulin must be replaced in a physiologic manner, and food intake and exercise must be carefully regulated in accord with the insulin prescription. An individualized meal plan designed to achieve and maintain normal weight and growth is critical. Generally, the meal plan contains approximately 50–55% of calories as carbohydrate, 15–20% as protein, and 30% as fat. Saturated fat and cholesterol are limited, fiber is encouraged, and instruction on postprandial glucose excursions from the intake of various types and amounts of carbohydrate is important. At least 3 meals with a bedtime snack are provided, with between-meal

219

snacks often recommended. Exercise must be timed and planned in advance and preferably should occur at least 5 days weekly at a set time.

Insulin is replaced either by insulin pump or by combining a basal insulin supply with premeal bolus injections. For intensive glycemic management, a type 1 diabetic patient usually has a total insulin requirement of 0.6–0.7 U/kg body weight on a daily basis. From 50–60% of this total dose is given as basal insulin and the remainder as rapid-acting insulin injected just before each meal. With an insulin pump, either lispro or aspart insulin is used. The basal rate may be set at a constant rate, or it may be programmed for variable rates for certain needs (such as an increase for the dawn phenomenon or a decrease during exercise). Premeal boluses are adjusted according to premeal blood glucose levels, calculated carbohydrate intake and portion size. Periodic check in of 1–2 hour postprandial and glucose levels will aid intensive management decisions.

The same principles are followed for type 1 diabetics managed by multiple insulin injections. Intensive management requires at least 3 or 4 injections daily, with glucose monitoring at each injection, to achieve the goals of fasting glucose levels of 80–120mg/dl and HbA1c <7%. Long-acting insulin should be used as the basal insulin replacement. Insulin glargine at bedtime is an excellent option, at an initial dose of about 0.3 U/kg in most patients. Dosage is adjusted to result in FBG levels of 80–120mg/dl before breakfast. Premeal lispro or aspart insulin is preferred (and is prescribed as in pump use) to make up the remainder of the 0.6–0.7 U/kg total 24-hour insulin requirement. A second option for basal insulin is to use ultralente, divided into two equal doses at breakfast and supper (total: 0.3 U/kg). In this method, rapid acting lispro or aspart can be mixed with ultralente and immediately injected before breakfast and supper. A separate injection of rapid acting insulin is used to cover lunch. Obviously, there will be individual variations in this general scheme because of different insulin sensitivities, variations in exercise and/or conditioning, meals, emotional stress, infections, and many other factors. With frequent contact with the health care team, most patients with type 1 diabetes can achieve the goals of intensive glycemic management.

Guidelines for Care

A compelling rationale is to have a goal of achieving normal levels of key clinical and biochemical markers. Fortunately, this goal of "normalcy" can be defended on the basis of large-scale, prospective clinical trials. In some systems, an action level is set, which is typically modestly greater than the normal goal. Although some may find this useful, others simply want to know the goal to strive for, with recognition that it may not always be possible to achieve. In diabetes, this is particularly true in the case of glycemic regulation, in which severe hypoglycemia (requiring the assistance of others) may be a serious limiting factor. This is particularly true for type 1 diabetes and is the major reason that the HbA1c goal is set at < 7%, instead of at the top normal for most laboratories of 6%. With this introduction, the goals of therapy in type 1 diabetes are as follows:

Assessment	Frequency	Goal
Diabetic education	Based on assessment	Understanding diabetes
Medical nutrition therapy	Based on assessment	Optimal weight
HbA1c	Twice yearly*	< 7%
Cholesterol	Yearly*	< 200 mg/dl
LDL-C	Yearly*	<100 mg/dl
HDL-C	Yearly*	> 45 mg/dl(M)
		> 55 mg/dl(F)
Triglyceride	Yearly*	< 150 mg/dl
Dilated eye exam	Yearly†	Prevent progression
Blood pressure	Each visit	< 130/80 mmHg
Urinary albumin	Yearly*†	< 30 mg/24 hr
Foot exam	Each Visit	Prevent amputation
Smoking assessment	Yearly	Prevent cardiovascular events
Aspirin therapy‡	Daily	Prevent cardiovascular events

*Quarterly if on drug therapy, until at goal.
†Except type 1 diabetes <10 yrs of age or within 5 years of diagnosis.
‡Over age 30; high cardiovascular risk.

Special Issues

Nephropathy

Microalbuminuria (> 30 mg/24 hours) is the first sensitive clinical indicator of diabetic nephropathy. Progression to clinical albuminuria (> 300 mg albumin/24 hours) is delayed or prevented by intensive glucose management and control of blood pressure to the goal of < 130/80 mmHg. ACE inhibitors and/or angiotensin receptor blockers are the agents of first choice and delay progression to end stage renal disease in patients with clinical proteinuria and elevated serum creatinine levels.

Hypertension

An elevation of blood pressure to ≥130/80 mmHg usually occurs in type 1 diabetes just before or at the time of development of microalbuminuria. At the stage of clinical albuminuria (urinary albumin > 300 mg/day), the majority of people with type 1 diabetes have BP levels > 130/80 mmHg. Aggressive therapy for hypertension should start at 130/80 mmHg to prevent progression of retinopathy, nephropathy, and cardiovascular events. As the duration of hypertension in type 1 diabetes lengthens, there is usually a need for more than one antihypertensive agent to maintain BP at the level of < 130/80 mmHg. Many specialists prefer to start with a low dose of an ACE inhibitor or angiotensin receptor blocker; add a low dose of a thiazide; add a low dose of a calcium channel blocker; and finally, add a low dose of a cardiospecific beta blocker. If this regimen does not bring BP to the goal of therapy, doses of each agent are then raised in a stepwise fashion until goal of < 130/80 mmHg is reached.

There are many variations on this scheme. Whatever approach is used, the evidence is strong that ACE inhibitor and/or ARB therapy must be used and that persistent adjustments are often necessary to achieve BP goals in type 1 diabetic patients with nephropathy and hypertension.

Lipids/Lipoproteins

When type 1 diabetes is reasonably well controlled on insulin therapy and the recommended diets, plasma lipid/lipoprotein levels are usually within normal limits. Albuminuria is the most common factor associated with an atherogenic lipid profile: elevated levels of plasma cholesterol; small, dense particles of LDL; and elevated plasma triglyceride levels with low HDL-C levels. If untreated, a persistent profile of this type is a major contributor to the increased risk of cardiovascular disease in type 1 diabetes. Other risk factors, such as hypertension, smoking, and hyperglycemia are also contributory. A standard of care, therefore is to monitor lipid/lipoprotein levels yearly and to institute statin therapy to an LDL-C goal of < 100 mg/dl. Fibrate therapy is used if triglyceride and HDL-C levels are not at their optimal levels. Niacin therapy is an option.

Retinopathy

Although intensive glycemic control is a major factor in preventing or delaying progression of diabetic retinopathy, other factors may also be operative in type 1 diabetes. In particular, hypertension accelerates progression of retinopathy, and aggressive therapy prevents progression. There may be a specific effect of ACE inhibitor therapy on retinopathy that is not mediated solely through blood pressure reduction. Yearly eye examinations by an eye specialist are indicated.

Pregnancy

There is no question that intensive glycemic management is necessary for excellent outcomes of pregnancy in type 1 diabetes. Ideally, the intensive program should start before conception and continue until delivery. It is best handled by alternating visits to the diabetes and obstetrics specialists, with increasing frequency often invoked as pregnancy progresses. Insulin requirements may transiently decrease in the first trimester, but then increase as pregnancy progresses, particularly in the third trimester. At delivery of the placenta, there is a rapid fall in requirements, usually to preconception levels. Regular ophthalmologic surveillance is needed, because retinopathy may progress during pregnancy. Monitoring of BP and urinary albumin are also indicated to recognize preeclampsia or the development of nephropathy.

Aspirin

Aspirin therapy is indicated for some but not all patients with type 1 diabetes. There are limited data about people under age 30, and Reye's syndrome can be an issue in younger patients. However, type 1 diabetic patients age 30 or older who are at high risk for cardiovascular events are candidates for aspirin therapy. High-risk patients are defined as those with strong family history of coronary heart disease, cigarette use, hypertension, albuminuria, BMI > 27 kg/m^2, or altered lipid/lipoprotein profile (mg/dl: cholesterol > 200, LDL-C > 100, triglycerides > 150, and/or HDL-C < 45 (men) or < 55 (women). Many patients have hypertension and/or indicators of diabetic nephropathy.

Flow Sheet

Every type 1 diabetic patient who is under intensive management for glycemia and other micro- and macrovascular risk factors should have a serial flow sheet. Computerized systems are available. Reference to the flow sheet before and during patient visits is an effective way to keep preventive management and the regular evaluations current. The flow sheet is also an excellent tool for discussing with each patient the goals of therapy, their rationale, and the success in achieving them.

Type 2 Diabetes

Pathophysiology and Natural History

Type 2 diabetes results in genetically susceptible people from insulin resistance and diminished insulin secretion by the pancreas. Loss of first-phase insulin secretion after a glucose stimulus is the first recognizable pancreatic functional defect. Postnutrient hyperglycemia occurs, and the pancreas secretes an excess of insulin in an attempt to return plasma glucose to or toward normal. In this phase of type 2 diabetes, impaired glucose tolerance is usually demonstrated. Over time, insulin output by the pancreas diminishes, and at the time of diagnosis by fasting hyperglycemia, insulin secretion is approximately 50% of normal. With increasing duration of type 2 diabetes, further diminution of insulin secretion occurs, hepatic glucose output increases, and insulin resistance of muscle, fat, and liver is accentuated by "glucose toxicity."

This sequence of events can be viewed as occurring in four stages

(Fig. 2, Chapter 8). In stage 1, diminished first-phase insulin secretion and impaired glucose tolerance may be managed by oral drugs that stimulate an immediate insulin release. Insulin resistance can be addressed by an intensive diet and exercise program and by insulin-sensitizing drugs. As the disease progresses, combination therapy that addresses the dual issues of diminished insulin secretion and insulin resistance are indicated. Combination therapy with insulin stimulators (meglitinides or sulfonylureas) and insulin sensitizers (metformin, thiazolidinediones) is needed. Triple oral therapy with an insulin stimulator, a thiazolidinedione to increase insulin sensitivity, and metformin to inhibit hepatic glucose output may be effective. Some physicians advocate adding an alpha glucosidase inhibitor to blunt the absorption of dietary carbohydrates. Thus, serial addition of many oral antidiabetic agents to address the diabetic state is feasible. The final step is insulin therapy, which can be used as basal replacement with continued oral agent therapy or as the sole pharmacologic agent. Guidelines for glycemic regulation are the same as in type 1 diabetes: the goal for fasting blood glucose is 80–120 mg/dl. Action should be taken for HbA1c > 8%, with a goal of < 7%.

In type 2 diabetes, hyperglycemia appears to be a major contributor to the progression of retinopathy, albuminuria, and neuropathy. In this respect, the main cause of the so-called "microvascular" complications of type 2 diabetes is comparable to type 1 diabetes. In both cases, prospective randomized trials have provided strong support for a policy of lowering HbA1c to as close to normal as safely possible. For every 1% lowering of an elevated HbA1c, there is about a 25% decrease in the risk for progression of diabetic retinopathy.

Cardiovascular Disease

Type 2 diabetes is characterized by accelerated cardiovascular disease. The risk for myocardial infarction, cardiovascular death, strokes, and peripheral vascular insufficiency is increased at least 2- to 4-fold in people with type 2 diabetes. These risks are doubled in African, Hispanic, and Mexican Americans and are magnified in a profound way by hypertension, dyslipidemia, cigarette smoking, and a prothrombotic state, which often is seen in type 2 diabetes. In particular, before the appearance of fasting hyperglycemia, many type 2 patients have had years of a metabolic syndrome, which confers a high cardiovascular risk. In this syndrome, glucose intolerance may be mild (or absent), but hypertension, microalbuminuria, low plasma HDL-C and high triglyceride levels, increased concentrations of atherogenic small, dense LDL particles, altered platelet function, diminished fibrinolytic activity and insulin resistance with hyperinsulinemia are present in various combinations. The net effect is that people with type 2 diabetes have a high cardiovascular risk from a variety of factors that are active even before fasting hyperglycemia and frank diabetes are apparent. Thus, a program of prevention of progression of accelerated atherothrombosis, which starts even before the diagnosis of type 2 diabetes is made, is the hallmark of intensive management of type 2 diabetes. A multifactorial approach that not only includes intensive glycemic regulation but also aggressively addresses multiple cardiovascular risk factors is indicated.

The goals of therapy are the same as in type 1 diabetes (see previous section). However, testing and preventive therapy for accelerated cardiovascular disease must proceed at an earlier stage in type 2 than in type 1 diabetes. Much of the evidence in support of aggressive cardiovascular risk reduction strategies in diabetes come from studies in type 2 diabetes (see below):

CV Risk Marker	Goal of Therapy	Preferred Agent(s)	Studies
Hypertension	< 130/80 mmHg	ACE inhibitor, ARB β-B, CCB, HCTZ	UKPDS, Syst-Eur, HOT, SHEP
↑ LDL-C	< 100 mg/dl	Statins	HPS, 4S, CARE
↓ HDL-C	≥ 45 mg/dl (men) ≥ 55 mg/dl (women)	Fibrates	VA-HIT, DAIS
↑ Triglycerides	< 150 mg/dl	Fibrates	VA-HIT, DAIS
↑ Platelet thromboxane	Inhibit	Aspirin	USPHS, ETDRS, HOT, APT
Angiotensin II	Inhibit	ACE inhibitor, ARB	HOPE, nephropathy studies

The studies and their references are given in Chapter 10.

Pertinent Web Sites

1. American Association of Diabetes Educators
   http://www.aadenet.org
2. American Diabetes Association
   http://www.diabetes.org
3. American Dietetic Association
   http://www.eatright.org
4. American Heart Association
   http://www.americanheart.org
5. American Society of Hypertension
   http://www.ash-us.org
6. Canadian Diabetes Association
   www.diabetes.ca
7. Center for Disease Control and Prevention
   http://www.cdc.gov/diabetes/index.htm
8. Diabetes in Control
   http://www.diabetesincontrol.com
9. Diabetes Initiative of South Carolina
   http://www.musc.edu/diabetes
10. European Association for the Study of Diabetes (EASD)
    http:www.easd.org
11. Juvenile Diabetes Research Foundation International
    http://jdf.org/index.php
12. Lipid Health
    http://www.lipidhealth.org
13. National Diabetes Education Program
    http://ndep.nih.gov
14. National Institutes of Health: NIDDK
    http://niddk.nih.gov

Index